Practical Biostatistics
A User-Friendly Approach for
Evidence-Based Medicine

Mendel Suchmacher
Professor of Clinical Immunology,
Carlos Chagas Institute of Medical Post-graduation,
Rio de Janeiro, Brazil

Mauro Geller
Professor and Chairman of Clinical Immunology,
Carlos Chagas Institute of Medical Post-graduation,
Rio de Janeiro, Brazil

AMSTERDAM • BOSTON • HEIDELBERG • LONDON
NEW YORK • OXFORD • PARIS • SAN DIEGO
SAN FRANCISCO • SINGAPORE • SYDNEY • TOKYO
Academic Press is an imprint of Elsevier

Academic Press is an imprint of Elsevier
32 Jamestown Road, London NW1 7BY, UK
225 Wyman Street, Waltham, MA 02451, USA
525 B Street, Suite 1800, San Diego, CA 92101-4495, USA

First edition 2012

Notice
No responsibility is assumed by the publisher for any injury and/or damage to
persons or property as a matter of products liability, negligence or otherwise, or from any
use or operation of any methods, products, instructions or ideas contained in the material
herein. Because of rapid advances in the medical sciences, in particular, independent veri-
fication of diagnoses and drug dosages should be made.

Trademarks/Registered Trademarks
Brand names mentioned in this book are protected by their respective trademarks and are
acknowledged.

British Library Cataloguing-in-Publication Data
A catalogue record for this book is available from the British Library

Library of Congress Cataloging-in-Publication Data
A catalog record for this book is available from the Library of Congress

ISBN: 978-0-12-415794-1

For information on all Academic Press publications
visit our website at elsevierdirect.com

Typeset by MPS Limited, Chennai, India
www.adi-mps.com

Printed and bound in United States of America

12 13 14 15 16   10 9 8 7 6 5 4 3 2 1

Contents

Part IV
Additional Concepts in Biostatistics

Our increasing awareness of biological mechanisms that underlie disease has vastly increased the possibility of performing clinical trials, epidemiological studies, and tests of new approaches to diagnosis and treatment. This, in turn, raises a major need for the investigator to understand the statistical principles that underlie the design, execution, and data analysis related to clinical research studies. Dr. Suchmacher and Dr. Geller have provided a practical and highly approachable guide to biostatistics in their book *Practical Biostatistics*. The first section will guide the reader through the steps involved in clinical trial design, including design principles, sample size calculation, choosing the most appropriate test, and hypothesis testing. The presentation is both concise and highly pragmatic, and includes self-evaluation questions with annotated answers. The other sections cover a variety of biostatistical issues, such as association studies, benefit-risk analysis, evaluation of diagnostic tests, approaches to meta-analysis, and correlation and regression analysis.

Although this book will not substitute for the need to collaborate with colleagues who have formal training in biostatistics, it will go a long way towards preparing the clinical investigator to design and carry out better studies. It will also prepare the investigator to work more productively with biostatistical experts. This book answers a real need in clinical research, and will be a welcome addition to the training armamentarium for clinical investigators.

Bruce Korf
Wayne H. and Sara Crews Finley
Professor of Medical Genetics
Chair, Department of Genetics
University of Alabama at Birmingham
USA

Preface

Clinical research has been evolving worldwide at an accelerated pace, over the last 30 years. The growing number of published papers, motivated by postgraduate programs or sponsored by official research incentive programs or pharmaceutical companies, is paralleled by regulatory demands based on sound scientific quality standards, considered undetachable from their ethical nature.

Even though engaged healthcare professionals and students, as well as professional clinical researchers, strive to accomplish the high technical skills demanded, some of them face difficulties in mastering biostatistics tools. These tools are necessary to critically interpret and assess papers already published, as well as to correctly develop and publish their own.

Driven by our own professional demands, we have been facing the challenge of assimilating mathematical concepts through Biostatistics-specialized literature, personal guidance, and clinical trials reading. Over the years, we continually documented the lessons learned until we reached the point where we noticed we had accumulated a significant body of knowledge, shareable with our colleagues. We then decided to organize, review (with the aid of a biostatistician) and publish it. By providing the project with Microsoft Office's Excel 2010 resources, we were able to propose a bridge between Biostatistics and the common technology user.

Obviously, we do not mean to exhaust the subject through this publication, but simply to make a didactic reference available to all professionals committed to the development of healthcare sciences who need to assimilate Biostatistical knowledge. Let them know this source was written by healthcare professionals just like them, who face the same difficulties as theirs. As a consequence, they are able to better interpret the literature necessary to compose their own studies, improve communication with the supporting biostatistician, and present their research as proficiently as possible.

We hope we achieved our goal, and that this modest contribution might be helpful to our readers.

Mendel Suchmacher
Mauro Geller

Acknowledgments

My mother, for taking me by the hand up to the point I could go on with my own feet.

My wife Ester and my son Renan, who accepted sacrificing our shared time so that this project could become a reality.

Luiz Claudio S. Brillanti and Renan Suchmacher, for their contribution to cover art and illustrations.

Joshua Dahlben (NYU) for language review of the manuscript.

Our patients, the very reason this book came into existence.

Introduction

The objective of Part I is to instruct the reader on how to choose the study type that best fits his or her research goals and material resources as well as how to determine the study type of a given paper.

Study Type Determination

A crucial stage in research planning is to determine the most suitable study type, according to the investigator's hypothesis (Chapter 4) and material resources available. A proposed classification of study types for epidemiological and clinical research is detailed in this chapter.

1.1 EPIDEMIOLOGICAL STUDIES

Epidemiological studies aim to establish the frequency of a condition in a given population. In this type of study, establishing reliable risk or etiological correlations is not possible because precise consistency between risk factors exposure or nonexposure, as well as between affected or nonaffected groups, cannot be achieved. For this reason, epidemiological studies remain mostly limited to measuring frequencies. Suspected risk correlations should be clarified through analytical studies.

Epidemiological studies can be classified into three types: ecological studies, cross-sectional studies, and longitudinal studies.

1.1.1 Ecological Studies

Ecological studies aim to determine the frequency of a given condition, supposedly associated with some environmental factor, during parallel or subsequent past time spans. For example, during the past 3 years, students from school A, which is located in an underprivileged district, have been presenting a higher frequency of upper respiratory virus infection compared to students from school B, which is located in a middle-class district, whose frequency is considered usual.

1.1.2 Cross-Sectional Studies

In cross-sectional studies, the frequency of a given condition in a naturally evolving population under a suspected exposure factor is analyzed, like a snapshot (Figure 1.1).

M. Suchmacher & M. Geller: Practical Biostatistics. DOI: 10.1016/B978-0-12-415794-1.00001-X

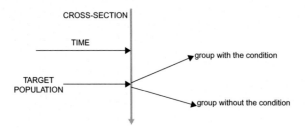

FIGURE 1.1   Schematic representation of cross-sectional study type.

1.1.3 Longitudinal Studies

In longitudinal studies, a cohort is followed for several years, or sometimes decades, in order to establish the frequencies of specific conditions and their correlation with environmental or other biological factors. Comparisons can be performed intrasubject or between different subjects, if possible. A classic example is the Framingham Heart Study, which began in 1948 with 5209 subjects and is currently in its third generation of participants. Knowledge on important environmental factors currently associated with cardiovascular risk, such as lifestyle (smoking, diet, and exercise) and aspirin use, has been derived from this study.

1.2 ANALYTICAL STUDIES

Analytical studies aim to establish correlation strength between a condition and a factor putatively associated with its origin and/or natural history. These types of studies are the main focus of this book and can be classified either as observational or intervention studies.

1.2.1 Observational Studies

In observational studies, the frequency of a condition in a population is studied under so-called "natural" circumstances. As such, active intervention from the investigator on these circumstances is not applicable. The main objective of observational studies is to establish the degree of hazard for a certain condition in relation to a considered exposure factor. Submitting the observed population to "real world" situations is its advantage. Its limitation is that it yields less accurate conclusions because uncontrolled variables and potential confounders may generate bias. Observational studies can be classified as case−control or cohort studies.

Case−Control Studies

In case−control studies, two groups are retrospectively compared, according to the following model: (1) One group with the condition (case) is subdivided into two subgroups — one exposed and the other nonexposed to a studied exposure factor; and (2) another group without the condition (control) is subdivided into two subgroups — one exposed and the other nonexposed to the same factor (Figure 1.2).

Case—control studies aim to determine the odds of acquiring a condition under exposure to a considered factor. For example, the odds of miners presenting asbestos-associated lung fibrosis relative to the general population are 1.5:1. The advantages of case—control studies are that they are less expensive to perform compared to cohort studies and they can be performed immediately because they are generally retrospective. Also due to this latter aspect, their limitations are: poor control over the exposure factor, uncontrolled variables, and potential confounders. Given the fact they focus on the outcome and "move back" toward the exposure factor, they are generally retrospective. Their inferred association strength — the odds ratio — is calculated using a specific formula (Chapter 2).

Cohort Studies

In cohort studies, a cohort of healthy subjects is divided into two groups according to exposure or nonexposure to a given factor — exposed subjects and nonexposed subjects — in principle for prospective follow-up. At the end of the study, the number of subjects with and without the condition is measured (Figure 1.3).

Cohort studies aim to determine the risk of acquiring a condition under exposure to a considered factor. For example, nuclear power plant workers have a 2.5 times greater risk of presenting high-grade lymphoma relative to nonexposed subjects. The advantage of these studies is that they afford better control over exposure level, covariates, and potential confounders because they are prospective. Their limitations are the need to wait for exposure factors to exert their effects and higher cost. Given the fact they focus on the exposure factor and "move forward" to the outcome, they are generally prospective.

Their inferred association strength — relative risk — is calculated using a specific formula (see Chapter 2). Note that the expression "cohort study" refers to a specific type of observational study. In this sense, the term "cohort" must be differentiated from its broader sense (see Glossary), which can be applied more widely.

Retrospective Cohort Studies

In retrospective cohort studies, two groups are retrospectively identified and "prospectively" compared according to the following model: A cohort of healthy subjects is subdivided into two groups — one exposed to a given factor and the other nonexposed to the same factor (Figure 1.4).

The advantages of retrospective cohort studies are that they are less expensive to perform than cohort studies and they can be performed immediately

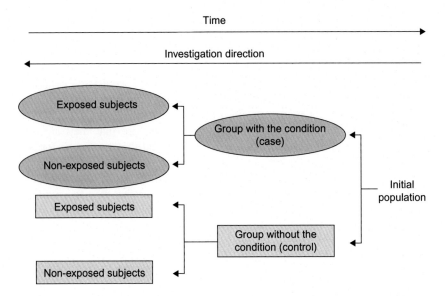

FIGURE 1.2   Schematic representation of a case−control study type.

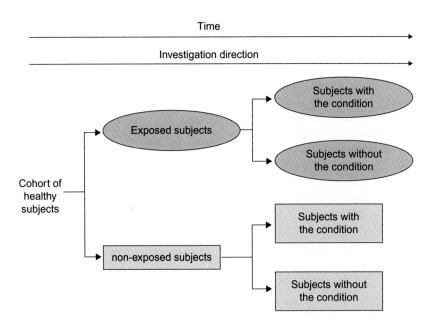

FIGURE 1.3   Schematic representation of a cohort study type.

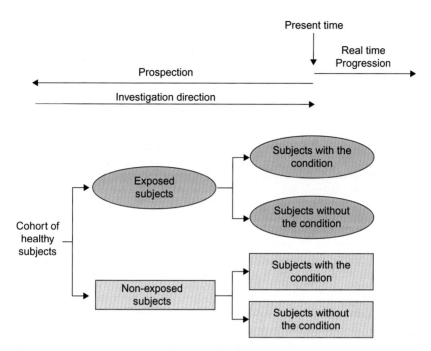

FIGURE 1.4   Graphic representation of a retrospective cohort study type.

because they are retrospective. Also due to this latter aspect, their limitation is: poor control over the exposure factor, covariates, and potential confounders.

1.2.2 Intervention Studies

Intervention studies (sometimes referred to as "randomized studies" or "controlled studies") are prospective cohort studies generally performed using a reference group (control group). Here, the investigator plans and actively intervenes with the factors influencing his or her cohort, minimizing the influence of uncontrolled variables and potential confounders. These studies are classified according to the applied intervention model.

Reference Standard

A study's reference standard changes according to its type: either noncomparative or comparative (controlled) studies.

Noncomparative Studies

In noncomparative studies, there is no reference standard to compare with the tested group. Results interpretation is difficult because the investigator can never be certain whether or not the findings represent an actual influence from the tested drug or vaccine.

Comparative Studies (Controlled Studies)

In comparative studies, there is a reference standard group (control) to compare to the tested group. The reference group is represented either by an active drug or vaccine known to be efficacious (active or positive control) or by placebo (negative control). Results interpretation by the investigator is more consistent because there is a comparison reference. In most situations, control group subjects are contemporary to tested group subjects. However, in some circumstances, historical (literature) controls can be used.

Relation Between Samples and Within Samples

The linkage between and within samples can change according to the study.

Nonpaired (Independent) Samples Studies

In nonpaired samples studies, individuals from a group can be freely matched for comparison with any individuals from the other group. Comparability is provided by the study design. For example, a sample of elderly patients admitted for cholelithiasis is divided into a group directed for emergency cholecystectomy and another group directed for conservative cholelithiasis management aiming for further elective surgery, and mortality and morbidity rates are compared.

Paired (Dependent) Samples Studies

In paired samples studies, individuals from a group can be matched for comparison exclusively with specific individuals from the other group. Three types of pairing are possible:

- Self-pairing: An individual is matched with him- or herself. For example, a sample of male patients with chronic neuropathic pain due to lumbar disk herniation complicated with radiculoneuropathy is treated with acupuncture for 3 months and with anticonvulsants for 3 months thereafter for optimal pain management comparison.
- Natural pairing: Natural pairing is performed between two different but extremely well linked individuals, such as monozygotic twins.
- Artificial pairing: Artificial pairing is performed between independent individuals, with pairing done according to a specific studied variable. For example, a sample of elderly patients admitted for cholelithiasis is divided into a group directed for emergency cholecystectomy and another group directed for conservative cholelithiasis management aiming for further elective surgery, and mortality and morbidity rates are compared. Nevertheless, according to study design, individuals from a group can

only be paired with individuals from the other group who share the same serum bilirubin level ranges.

Awareness of Tested Drug, Vaccine, or Exam

Open studies, single-blind studies and double-blind studies have different levels of awareness, either from the investigator or the study subject, or both.

Open Studies

In open studies, both the investigator and the study subject are aware of the nature of the tested drug or vaccine. It is applied whenever it is neither possible nor desirable to conceal them from both. An example is a comparison study between PUVA (psoralen + UVA exposure) and subcutaneous etanercept for skin psoriasis control. The limitation of open studies is bias generation both from the investigator and from the study subject.

Single-Blind Studies

In single-blind studies, the investigator, but not the study subject, is aware of the tested drug or vaccine. It is applied whenever it is neither possible nor advisable for the investigator to not be aware of them. An example is a comparison study between dobutamine and milrinone efficacy for pulmonary capillary wedge pressure control during cardiogenic shock. The limitation of single-blinded studies is bias generation due to self-suggestion by the investigator.

Double-Blind Studies

In double-blind studies, neither the investigator nor the study subject are aware of the tested drug or vaccine. It is applied to avoid bias generation due to self-suggestion from both parties. An example is a comparison study between placebo and a type 5 phosphodiesterase inhibitor for erectile dysfunction management.

Study Subject Allocation Method

The allocation method for the study can be either nonrandomized or randomized.

Nonrandomized Studies

In nonrandomized studies, the investigator selects study subjects to be allocated to one of the study groups according to pre-established criteria. It is applied whenever study design demands selective allocation. An example is an influenza vaccine efficacy study of two groups of subjects of different age ranges (40−50 and 60−70 years). Nonrandomized studies are susceptible to bias due to misinterpretation of data.

Randomized Studies

In randomized studies, the investigator randomly allocates study subjects into study groups. The advantages of these studies are:

- Random error minimization through equal distribution of individual characteristics between or among study groups.
- Systematic error minimization through avoidance of study subject selectivity by the investigator.
- Minimization of the influence of uncontrolled variables through equal distribution between or among study groups.

Follow-Up Methods

Follow-up methods for a study can include parallel or crossover studies.

Parallel Studies

In parallel studies, study groups progress in parallel during the investigation until its end.

Crossover Studies

In crossover studies, the groups change their respective arms at a specific point during the investigation. For example, a new ergot alkaloid derivative+ acetaminophen combination showed a significant decrease in migraine symptoms in group A subjects compared to group B subjects, who took only acetaminophen. After regimen swap, group B subjects showed the same symptom decrease first associated with group A subjects, and the latter presented the same symptoms level that group B subjects did in the first phase of the study. Advantages of crossover studies are:

- They corroborate the findings of the first phase of the study by reproducing them in the second phase, reinforcing the final conclusion of the study.
- They afford comparison between groups in a self-paired manner; that is, groups A and B can be compared against themselves at the end of the study, and this allows for greater biological homogeneity.

The limitation of crossover studies is the need for a washout period between study phases.

Study design is the combination of the awareness level of the tested drug or vaccine, the chosen comparative reference, study subject allocation and follow-up methods, the planned duration of the study, the number of groups and subgroups, and the exams involved — all adjusted to provide an answer to the investigator's hypothesis. A randomized, double-blind, crossover, placebo-controlled trial is an example of a desirable study design.

1.3 SUMMARY OF STUDY TYPES

The following classification is not definitive. Different study types not listed and study types in which mixed characteristics are adopted can be implemented depending on the investigator's objectives and resources.

- Epidemiological studies
  - Ecological studies
  - Cross-sectional studies
  - Longitudinal studies
- Analytical studies
  - Observational studies
    - Case−control studies
    - Cohort studies
    - Retrospective cohort studies
  - Intervention studies
    - Reference standard
       Noncomparative studies
       Comparative studies
    - Relation between samples and within samples
       Nonpaired sample studies
       Paired sample studies
          Self-pairing
          Natural pairing
          Artificial pairing
    - Awareness of tested drug or vaccine
       Open studies
       Single-blind studies
       Double-blind studies
    - Study subjects allocation method
       Nonrandomized studies
       Randomized studies
    - Follow-up method
       Parallel studies
       Crossover studies

Study type choice will aid in the decision-making process to determine the most appropriate biostatistical model for answering the investigator's hypothesis.

Part I Reader Resources

SELF-EVALUATION

1. Find the correct correspondence:
     1. Comparative studies
     2. Artificial pairing
     3. Randomization
     4. Crossover
     5. Cross-sectional studies

     a. Pattern of relation of a studied sample with another sample
     b. A form of analyzing a condition frequency, used in epidemiological studies
     c. A type of reference standard used in intervention studies
     d. A follow-up method used in intervention studies
     e. A form of subject allocation in a study

   A. 1−b, 2−e, 3−c, 4−d, 5−a
   B. 1−c, 2−e, 3−a, 4−d, 5−b
   C. 1−c, 2−a, 3−e, 4−d, 5−b
   D. 1−a, 2−e, 3−d, 4−c, 5−b

2. Mark the incorrect affirmative:
   A. Cohort studies can only be prospective.
   B. Double-blind studies provide more reliable results than single-blind studies.
   C. Relative risk is an index that provides more robust information than odds ratio.
   D. In parallel studies, subjects from study groups can never be swapped.

3. Read the following study abstract and then answer the question:

With the aim of assessing the relation between C-section, vaginal delivery, and Apgar scoring in the obstetrics ward of a county hospital during a 10-year period, 2052 patient records were retrospectively evaluated. An Apgar ≤6 was considered as the cutoff score, and Apgar scores >6 were considered as the control. Premature infants and infants from mothers with reports of severe abnormalities during prenatal care were not included.

How would you classify this study?
   A. Randomized intervention study
   B. Double-blind comparative study
   C. Cohort study
   D. Case−control study

ANNOTATED ANSWERS

1. C.

2. A. In retrospective cohort studies, two groups are retrospectively identified and "prospectively" compared in a similar manner as in usual cohort studies.

3. D. The authors' statement implies that establishing some degree of relationship between C-section and vaginal delivery procedures and Apgar scoring is intended, and this excludes epidemiological studies. This study is not prospective, and this clearly excludes intervention studies as well. Observe the following diagram:

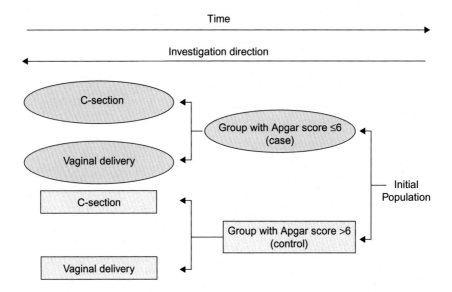

It can be seen that C-section and vaginal delivery groups were retrospectively followed as case (Apgar ≤6) and control (Apgar >6), and that they represented the "exposure" and "nonexposure" factors, respectively. Hence, this study can be classified as a case−control study type.

SUGGESTED READING

Basic statistics for clinicians, 1995. Can. Med. Assoc. J. <www.cmaj.ca>.

Estrela, C., 2001. Metodologia Científica: Ensino e Pesquisa em Odontologia. Editora Artes Médicas, Sao Paulo, Brazil.

Everitt, B., 2006. Medical Statistics from A to Z: A Guide for Clinicians and Medical Students, second ed. Cambridge University Press, Cambridge, UK.

Everitt, B.S., et al., 2005. Encyclopaedic Companion to Medical Statistics. Hodder Arnold, London.

Hulley, S.B., et al., 2001. Designing Clinical Research: An Epidemiological Approach, second ed. Lippincott Williams & Wilkins, Philadelphia.

Sackett, D.L., et al., 2001. Evidence-Based Medicine: How to Practice and Teach EBM, second ed. Churchill Livingstone, Edinburgh, UK.

Observational Studies

The objective of Part II is to expand the knowledge base on observational studies and to introduce derivative concepts: odds ratio, relative risk, and number needed to harm. Models for increasing the accuracy of this study type are also described.

Chapter 2

Determination of Association Strength between an Exposure Factor and an Event in Observational Studies

The aim in intervention studies is to demonstrate the difference — generally as a favorable outcome — between two groups. Alternatively, the goal in observational studies is to measure the odds or the risk for the occurrence of an event between two groups. Based on the observational study type, two different approaches are possible.

2.1 CASE–CONTROL STUDIES

Odds ratio (OR) is an index for association strength determination between an exposure factor and an event. In observational studies, it expresses the ratio between the odds for the occurrence of an event in a group exposed to a factor and the odds for the occurrence of the same event in a group exposed to a different factor (or not exposed). OR may be used in studies of epidemiological interest or in therapeutic observational studies. OR can also derive the number needed to harm (discussed later).

2.1.1 Odds Ratio

Odds Ratio for Studies of Epidemiological Interest

As an example, a population of 100 individuals is divided into a group with lung cancer (case) and a group without lung cancer (control), with the aim of measuring the odds for the occurrence of lung cancer related to smoke exposure. Both groups are divided into two subgroups—smokers and nonsmokers—and retrospectively followed for up to 25 years (Figure 2.1 and Table 2.1).

Based on the results, we can infer the following:

- There is 4:1 odds of smokers presenting lung cancer (*a/b*).
- There is 1:4 odds of nonsmokers presenting lung cancer (*c/d*).

M. Suchmacher & M. Geller: Practical Biostatistics. DOI: 10.1016/B978-0-12-415794-1.00002-1

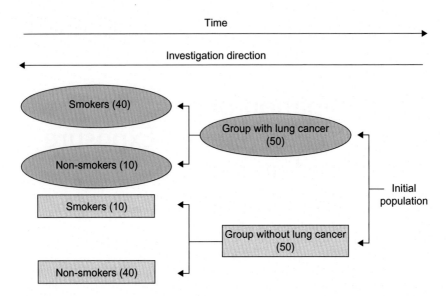

FIGURE 2.1 Schematic representation of an initial population of healthy and lung cancer patients, under a case−control study type.

TABLE 2.1 Study Results for Odds Ratio Calculation

| | Results | |
	Case	Control
Smokers	40 (*a*)	10 (*b*)
Nonsmokers	10 (*c*)	40 (*d*)

Establishing the Odds Ratio

$$OR = \frac{a/b}{c/d}$$

$$OR = \frac{40/10}{10/40} = 16$$

This result means that the odds of lung cancer occurrence is 16:1 for smokers in relation to nonsmokers.

Odds Ratio for Therapeutic Studies

As an example, a population of 120 perimenopaused women is divided into a group with perimenopausal symptoms (case) and a group without perimenopausal symptoms (control), with the aim of measuring the odds of the occurrence of perimenopausal symptoms relative to regular ingestion of soy isoflavones. The groups are each divided into two subgroups: subgroup A, comprising women who regularly ingest soy isoflavones, and subgroup B, comprising women who do not ingest soy isoflavones. Both groups are retrospectively followed for up to 10 years (Figure 2.2 and Table 2.2).

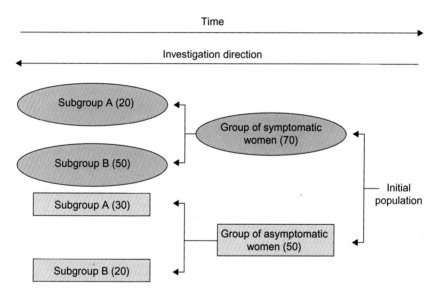

FIGURE 2.2   Schematic representation of a population of perimenopaused women, under a case−control study type.

TABLE 2.2 **Study Results for Odds Ratio Calculation**

	Results	
	Case	*Control*
Subgroup A	20 (*a*)	30 (*b*)
Subgroup B	50 (*c*)	20 (*d*)

Based on the results, we can infer the following:

- There is 0.6:1 odds of women who regularly ingest soy isoflavones presenting perimenopausal symptoms (*a/b*).
- There is 2.5:1 odds of women who do not ingest soy isoflavones presenting perimenopausal symptoms (*c/d*).

Establishing the Odds Ratio

$$OR = \frac{a/b}{c/d}$$

$$OR = \frac{20/30}{50/20} = 0.26$$

This result means that the odds of the occurrence of perimenopausal symptoms is 0.2:1 for women who regularly ingest soy isoflavones in relation to women who do not ingest soy isoflavones.

2.1.2 Number Needed to Harm

Number needed to harm (NNH) corresponds to the number of individuals who must be treated so that one individual presents an adverse reaction accountable to the treatment. The main usefulness of NNH is to make the OR data more practical to physicians and comprehensible for patients. Its interpretation must be performed based on the physician's practice experience and on NNHs established for other treatment modalities related to the case. For example, a population of 180 individuals with recently treated lung tuberculosis is divided into a group with drug-induced hepatitis (case) and a group without drug-induced hepatitis (control), with the aim of measuring the odds of the occurrence of isoniazid-related hepatitis. The groups are divided into two subgroups: regimen A, treated with isoniazid, and regimen B, not treated with isoniazid. Both groups are retrospectively followed until the beginning of tuberculostatic regimens (Figure 2.3 and Table 2.3).

$$OR = \frac{a/b}{c/d}$$

$$OR = \frac{65/35}{35/45} = 2.4$$

NNH is calculated using the following formula:

$$\frac{1 - [PEER \times (1 - OR)]}{(1 - PEER) \times PEER \times (1 - OR)}$$

where PEER is the patient expected event rate.

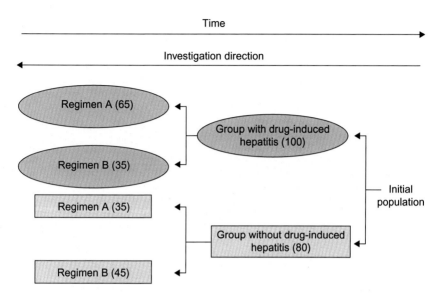

FIGURE 2.3   Schematic representation of a population of recently treated tuberculosis patients, under a case–control study type.

TABLE 2.3 Study Results for Odds Ratio Calculation

		Results	
Regimen A	65 (*a*)		35 (*b*)
Regimen B	35 (*c*)		45 (*d*)

In this example, the chosen PEER corresponds to the proportion of regimen B individuals belonging to the drug-induced hepatitis group: 30% (or 0.3).

$$\frac{1 - [0.3 \times (1 - 2.4)]}{(1 - 0.3) \times 0.3 \times (1 - 2.4)} = 5$$

This result means that it would be necessary to treat five patients with lung tuberculosis for one to present isoniazid drug-induced hepatitis.

Alternatively, it is possible to consult an NNH table (Tables 2.4 and 2.5).

2.1.3 Summary

Case–control studies allow group rather than individual-to-individual exposure assessment because they afford less control over study conditions. For this reason, this type of study does not allow for risk but, rather, odds status

TABLE 2.4 NNH Table for Odds Ratio Calculation < 1.0

		For OR < 1.0						
		0.9	*0.8*	*0.7*	*0.6*	*0.5*	*0.4*	*0.3*
PEER	0.05	209	104	69	52	41	34	29
	0.10	110	54	36	27	21	18	15
	0.20	61	30	20	14	11	10	8
	0.30	46	22	14	10	8	7	5
	0.40	40	19	12	9	7	6	4
	0.50	83	18	11	8	6	5	4
	0.70	44	10	13	9	6	5	4
	0.90	101	46	27	18	12	9	4

TABLE 2.5 NNH Table for Odds Ratio Calculation > 1.0

		For OR > 1.0						
		1.1	*1.25*	*1.5*	*1.75*	*2*	*2.25*	*2.5*
PEER	0.05	212	86	44	30	28	18	16
	0.10	113	46	24	16	13	10	9
	0.20	64	27	14	10	8	7	6
	0.30	50	21	11	8	7	6	5
	0.40	44	19	10	8	6	6	5
	0.50	42	18	10	8	6	6	5
	0.70	51	23	13	10	9	8	7
	0.90	121	55	33	25	22	19	18

correlations only. This also explains why OR has limited usefulness in intervention cohort studies.

Determination of OR values that suggest a significant relationship between the exposure factor and the event is empirically based. Normally, the following factors are taken into consideration:

- Influence of unknown variables and potential confounders: Case–control studies are more prone to the occurrence of unknown variables and

confounders than are cohort studies. Therefore, there is a higher "toler-ance" for the assumption of more elevated OR values.
- Event severity: The more severe the event, the lesser the "tolerance" for the assumption of more elevated OR values.

2.2 COHORT STUDIES

Relative risk (RR) is an index for association strength determination between an exposure factor and an event. It is defined as the ratio between the risk for the occurrence of an event in a group exposed to a factor and the risk for the occurrence of the same event in a group exposed to a different factor (or not exposed). RR may be used in studies of epidemiological interest or in therapeutic observational studies. By analogy with OR, RR can also derive the NNH.

2.2.1 Relative Risk

Relative Risk for Studies of Epidemiological Interest

As an example, a population of 100 individuals is divided into an exposed group (smokers) and a nonexposed group (nonsmokers), with the aim of measuring the risk for the occurrence of lung cancer related to smoke expo-sure. Both groups are prospectively followed for 15 years and then divided into two subgroups each − individuals with lung cancer and individuals without lung cancer (Figure 2.4 and Table 2.6).

Based on the results, we can infer the following:

- There is an 80% risk of smoke-exposed individuals presenting lung can-cer $[a/(a + b)]$.
- There is a 40% risk of non-smoke-exposed individuals presenting lung cancer $[c/(c + d)]$.

Establishing the Relation Between the Risks

$$RR = \frac{[a/(a + b)]}{[c/(c + d)]}$$

$$RR = \frac{[40/(40 + 10)]}{[20/(20 + 30)]} = 2$$

This result means that the risk of lung cancer is twice as high among smoke-exposed individuals in relation to nonexposed individuals.

Relative Risk for Therapeutic Studies

As an example, a population of 120 perimenopaused women is divided into group A (women who regularly ingest soy isoflavones) and group B (women

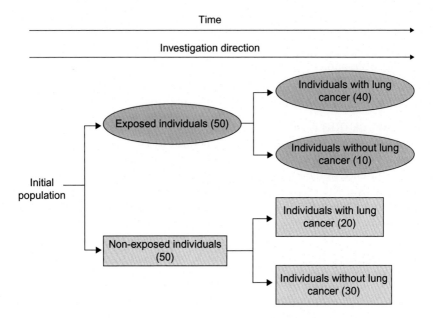

FIGURE 2.4 Schematic representation of a population of smoking-exposed and -nonexposed individuals, under a cohort study type.

TABLE 2.6 Study Results for Risk Calculation

	Results		
	With Lung Cancer	*Without Lung Cancer*	*Total*
Exposed	40 (*a*)	10 (*b*)	50
Nonexposed	20 (*c*)	30 (*d*)	50

who do not ingest soy isoflavones), with the aim of measuring the risk for the occurrence of perimenopausal symptoms relative to regular ingestion of soy isoflavones. Both groups are prospectively followed for 3 years and then divided into two subgroups each — symptomatic women and asymptomatic women (Figure 2.5 and Table 2.7).

Based on the results, we can infer the following:

- There is a 28% risk of women who regularly ingest soy isoflavones presenting perimenopausal symptoms [$a/(a + b)$].
- There is a 60% risk of women who do not ingest soy isoflavones presenting perimenopausal symptoms [$c/(c + d)$].

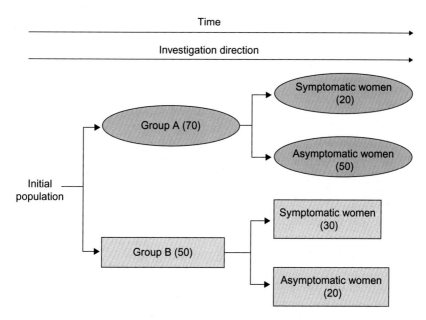

FIGURE 2.5   Schematic representation of a population of perimenopaused women, under a cohort study type.

TABLE 2.7 Study Results for RR Calculation

	Results		
	Symptomatic	Asymptomatic	Total
Group A	20 (a)	50 (b)	70
Group B	30 (c)	20 (d)	50

Establishing the Relation Between the Risks

$$RR = \frac{[a/(a+b)]}{[c/(c+d)]}$$

$$RR = \frac{[20/(20+50)]}{[30/(30+20)]} \cong 0.5$$

This result means that the risk of the occurrence of perimenopausal symptoms is 0.5 for women who regularly ingest soy isoflavones in relation to women who do not ingest soy isoflavones.

2.2.2 Number Needed to Harm

NNH corresponds to the number of individuals who must be treated so that one of them presents an adverse reaction accountable to the treatment. The main usefulness of NNH is to make RR data more practical to physicians and comprehensible for patients. Its interpretation must be performed based on physician's own practice experience and on NNHs established for other treatment modalities related to the case. For example, a population of 180 individuals with diagnosis of lung tuberculosis is divided into two groups treated with different regimens, with the aim of measuring the risk for the occurrence of isoniazid drug-induced hepatitis: regimen A, isoniazid included, and regimen B, isoniazid not included. Both groups are prospectively followed for 1 year and then divided into two subgroups each — individuals with drug-induced hepatitis and individuals without drug-induced hepatitis (Figure 2.6 and Table 2.8).

NNH is calculated using the following formula:

$$[a/(a+b)] - [c/(c+d)]$$
$$[65/(65+35)] - [35/(35+45)] = 0.22 \Rightarrow 22$$

This result means that it is necessary to treat 22 patients with lung tuberculosis so that one presents isoniazid drug-induced hepatitis.

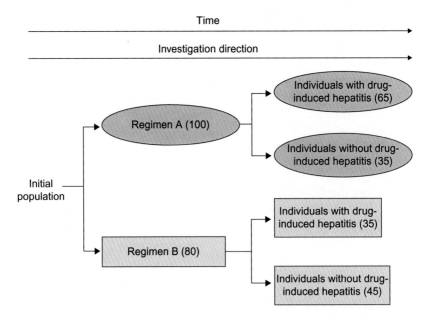

FIGURE 2.6   Schematic representation of a population of tuberculosis patients, under a cohort study type.

TABLE 2.8 Study Results for NNH Calculation

	Results		
	With Hepatitis	*Without Hepatitis*	*Total*
Regimen A	65 (*a*)	35 (*b*)	100
Regimen B	35 (*c*)	45 (*d*)	80

2.2.3 Summary

Cohort studies allow individual-to-individual rather than group exposure assessment because they afford more control over study conditions. For this reason, this type of study allows risk status correlations. An intervention study can also derive a cohort study if its adverse reaction results (often the endpoint for which RR is more useful in this type of study) are submitted to this kind of approach.

Determination of RR values that suggest a significant relationship between the exposure factor and the event is empirically based. Normally, two factors are taken into consideration:

- Influence of unknown variables and potential confounders: Cohort studies are less prone to the occurrence of unknown variables and confounders than are case–control studies. Therefore, there is a smaller tolerance for the assumption of more elevated RR values.
- Event severity: The more severe the event, the lesser the tolerance for the assumption of more elevated RR values.

Chapter 3

Increasing Accuracy in Observational Studies

An important limitation of observational studies is the poor control exerted by the investigator over study conditions, making the study subject susceptible to the effects of uncontrolled variables different from the major variable – condition or exposure. These uncontrolled variables either influence (prospective studies) or will have influenced (retrospective studies) the evolution of the study, making interpretation of results more difficult. However, it is possible to minimize this effect by including these uncontrolled variables on study protocol as covariates. Stratified analysis and multivariable analysis are two types of statistical resources used for this purpose.

3.1 STRATIFIED ANALYSIS

In stratified analysis, covariates different from the major variables – condition or exposure – are weighted in odds ratio (OR) and relative risk (RR) calculations, respectively. Through stratification of case/control and exposure/nonexposure groups, new data can be inferred (only bivariate analysis – that is, one covariate at a time against the major variable – is detailed). Let us use two examples from Chapter 4.

3.1.1 Example 1

A population of 120 perimenopaused women presented an OR of 0.26:1 for the occurrence of perimenopausal symptoms for women who regularly ingest soy isoflavones in relation to women who do not ingest soy isoflavones (see example from Section 2.1.1 in Chapter 2). General study results are detailed in Table 3.1.

$$OR = \frac{20/30}{50/20} = 0.26$$

M. Suchmacher & M. Geller: Practical Biostatistics. DOI: 10.1016/B978-0-12-415794-1.00003-3

TABLE 3.1 General Study Results for OR Calculation

| | Results | |
	Case	Control
Subgroup A	20	30
Subgroup B	50	20

TABLE 3.2 Study Results According to the 40- to 50-Year-Old Age Range

| | Results | |
	Case	Control
Subgroup A	3	16
Subgroup B	5	2

TABLE 3.3 Study Results According to the 51- to 65-Year-Old Age Range

| | Results | |
	Case	Control
Subgroup A	7	8
Subgroup B	15	3

Then, both subgroups are stratified according to the following age ranges:

- 40−50 years old (Table 3.2):

$$OR = \frac{3/10}{20/7} = 0.07$$

- 51−65 years old (Table 3.3):

$$OR = \frac{10/8}{10/6} = 0.17$$

- 66−80 years old (Table 3.4):

$$OR = \frac{7/12}{20/7} = 0.8$$

TABLE 3.4 Study Results According to the 66- to 80-Year-Old Age Range

	Results	
	Case	*Control*
Subgroup A	10	6
Subgroup B	30	15

TABLE 3.5 General Study Results for RR Calculation

	Results	
	With Lung Cancer	*Without Lung Cancer*
Exposed	40	10
Nonexposed	20	30

As can be clearly noticed, OR increases across the three proposed age ranges. Had we not performed this stratification, this important information would have remained undetected. Nevertheless, the hypothesis of whether these results should represent significant differences must be tested using statistical tests (see Chapter 9).

3.1.2 Example 2

A population of 100 individuals presented an RR of 2 for the occurrence of lung cancer related to smoke exposure for smokers in relation to nonsmokers (see example from Section 2.2.1 in Chapter 2). General study results are detailed in Table 3.5.

$$RR = \frac{[40/(40 + 10)]}{[20/(20 + 30)]} = 2$$

Then, both groups are stratified according to family history for lung cancer:

- Negative family history (Table 3.6):

$$RR = \frac{[22/(22 + 6)]}{[12/(12 + 16)]} = 1.8$$

- Positive family history (Table 3.7):

$$RR = \frac{[18/(18 + 4)]}{[8/(8 + 14)]} = 2.2$$

TABLE 3.6 Study Results According to a Positive Family History

	Results	
	With Lung Cancer	*Without Lung Cancer*
Exposed	22	6
Nonexposed	12	16

TABLE 3.7 Study Results According to a Negative Family History

	Results	
	With Lung Cancer	*Without Lung Cancer*
Exposed	18	4
Nonexposed	8	14

As can be clearly seen, RR differs according to a family history for lung cancer. Had we not performed this stratification, this important information would have remained undetected. Nevertheless, the hypothesis of whether these results should represent significant differences must be tested using statistical tests.

3.2 MULTIVARIABLE ANALYSIS

The reader is advised to study Chapter 14 before exploring this section.

Multivariable analysis represents a more robust tool for inaccuracy minimization in observational studies compared to stratified analysis. Through this approach, the effects of different covariates (independent variables) on study outcome (dependent variable) are first considered individually and then simultaneously for a more realistic result. Let us illustrate this concept using an example of a case−control study.

With the aim of determining the degree of influence from combined covariates (independent variables) on blood glucose level (dependent variable) abnormalities during the first 3 days in an adult postoperative intensive care unit (ICU), the records of 804 patients admitted to the ICU during a 3-year time span were retrospectively investigated. Blood glucose levels from 792 ICU patients, measured during their first 3 days of admission, served as controls.

Multiple linear regression was the type of multivariable analysis applied. Cutoffs for abnormal blood glucose levels were <50 and >140 mg/dL.

First, ORs were calculated for each covariate individually, regardless of the other coavariates (crude OR; calculations not shown). Then, multiple linear regression analysis was performed, when biological influence of study covariates on each other was weighted, for OR recalculation (adjusted OR; calculations not shown) (Table 3.8).

Crude OR results indicated age older than 65 years, orthopedic surgery, diagnosis of postoperative systemic inflammatory response syndrome/sepsis, and preoperative risk assessment as the covariates more strongly associated with abnormal blood glucose levels. After multivariable analysis, results are consistent with neurosurgery, use of insulin, and preoperative risk assessment as the covariates more strongly associated to this abnormality.

Multivariable analysis is robust enough to eventually identify some covariates as confounders because its methods can comprehend several covariates simultaneously. However, it cannot adjust for unknown variables. Only through randomization is it possible to compensate for their presence by evenly distributing them between or among groups.

TABLE 3.8 Crude OR and OR After Multivariable Analysis (Adjusted OR) of 7503 Observations Related to Abnormal Blood Glucose Levels in ICU Postoperative Patients and 6903 Observations Related to ICU Nonsurgical Patients

	Crude OR	Adjusted OR
Age >65 years	1.01*	1.02
Gender	1.3	1.0
Abdominal surgery	0.9	1.0
Orthopedic surgery	1.0*	0.8
Neurosurgery	1.0	1.3*
Diagnosis of preoperative infection	1.2	1.3
Diagnosis of postoperative SIRS/sepsis	1.3*	1.7
Use of adrenaline (y/n)	1.8	1.4
Use of insulin (y/n)	1.9	1.3*
Preoperative risk assessment	1.9*	2.0*

*Strength of association between the variable and blood glucose levels was statistically significant (p < 0.05).
SIRS, systemic inflammatory response syndrome.

Part II Reader Resources

SELF-EVALUATION

1. Analyze the following abstract of a case—control study and mark the incorrect affirmative:

   A sample of 112 radiotherapy technicians was subdivided into two groups — with and without diagnosis of a temporal condition — and retrospectively followed for 10 years. Frequency and duration of radiation exposure, as well as other present or past comorbidities and exposure to different risk factors, were evaluated using a questionnaire.

   A. Advantages of case—control studies are affordability and the possibility of immediate start-up.
   B. Case—control studies yield more reliable associations than do cohort studies because they use prospectively collected data.
   C. The odds of acquiring a tumoral condition could be quantified by the odds ratio in this case—control study.
   D. The odds of acquiring a condition under exposure to a considered factor can be quantified through case—control studies.

2. Read the following study abstract and then answer the question:

   The objective of this multicentric, case—control study was to determine the influence of hepatitis C virus infection on moderate to severe internal hemorrhage rates in hemophilia A patients. Medical records and death certificates of a sample of 3900 hemophilia A patients (2110 hepatitis C virus carriers and 1790 non-hepatitis C virus carriers) were analyzed, corresponding to a 5-year period. The following rates were found: (1) hepatitis C virus carriers group, 1106 moderate to severe internal hemorrhage episodes; and (2) non-hepatitis C virus carriers group, 830 moderate to severe hemorrhage episodes (OR, 1.27; p < 0.05).

   Mark the incorrect affirmative:
   A. Hemophilia A patients who did not present hemorrhage corresponded to the control group.
   B. In this sample of hemophilia A patients, individuals infected with hepatitis C virus had a 1.27 odds of presenting moderate to severe internal hemorrhage.
   C. In this sample of hemophilia A patients, individuals infected with hepatitis C virus had a 1.27 risk of presenting moderate to severe internal hemorrhage.
   D. This study is an observational type of study.

3. Read the following study abstract and then answer the question:

The primary objective of this cohort study was to measure the risk for cataract formation as a complication from prolonged topical corticosteroid use for chronic idiopathic anterior uveitis. A cohort of patients with a diagnosis of idiopathic chronic anterior uveitis of 3 years' duration (n = 96), followed in our institution, was randomized: (1) 52 patients to prednisolone 1% one drop q6h and (2) 44 patients to homatropine 2% one drop q3h, both administered in both eyes for a 1-year period. Visual acuity was the adopted endpoint, with 20/200 vision as cutoff for mature cataract staging. Lens opacity was confirmed by slit lamp examination. Results: 34 patients from the prednisolone group and 23 patients from the homatropine group showed evidence of mature cataract at the end of study. Conclusion: Prolonged topical prednisolone administration for chronic anterior uveitis significantly increased the risk for cataract formation in the studied population (p < 0.05).

    What is the number needed to harm (NNH) for the prolonged topical corticosteroid group, inferable from this study?
  A. 19
  B. 20
  C. 10
  D. 13

4. Mark the incorrect affirmative:
  A. Confounders are susceptible to identification by multivariable analysis.
  B. In stratified analysis of case−control and cohort studies, covariates different from condition or exposure are simultaneously weighted.
  C. Multivariable analysis cannot be adjusted for unknown variables in observational studies.
  D. Multivariable analysis is a more robust tool than stratified analysis for increasing accuracy of observational studies.

ANNOTATED ANSWERS

1. B. Actually, it is the opposite. Because cohort studies are prospective, they afford better planning and more strict control over study conditions than do case−control studies; therefore, they yield more reliable results.
2. C. Because case−control studies are basically retrospective, and therefore afford less control, they permit group rather than individual-to-individual exposure assessment. For this reason, this type of study does not afford risk but, rather, odds status correlations only.

3. D.

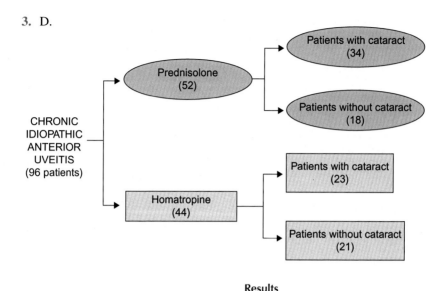

Results

	With Cataract	Without Cataract
Prednisolone	34 (a)	18 (b)
Homatropine	23 (c)	21 (d)

$$NNH = [(a/(a + b)] - [c/(c + d)]$$
$$[34/(34 + 18)] - [23/(23 + 21)] = 0.13 \Rightarrow 13$$

This result means that it would be necessary to treat 13 patients with chronic idiopathic anterior uveitis diagnosis under a prolonged topical corticosteroids regimen so that one of them presented cataract.

4. B. In stratified analysis, covariates are individually rather than simultaneously weighted.

SUGGESTED READING

Basic statistics for clinicians. Can. Med. Assoc. J. <www.cmaj.ca>.

Everitt, B.S., 1995. The Cambridge Dictionary of Statistics in the Medical Sciences. Cambridge, University Press, Cambridge.

Everitt, B.S., et al., 2005. Encyclopaedic Companion to Medical Statistics. Hodder Arnold, London.

Hulley, S.B., et al., 2001. Designing Clinical Research: An Epidemiological Approach, second ed. Lippincott Williams & Wilkins, Philadelphia.

Jaeschke, R., Guyatt, G., Shannon, H., Walter, S., Cook, D., Heddle, N., 1995. Assessing the effects of treatment: measures of association. Can. Med. Assoc. J. 152, 351−357.

Katz, M.H., 1999. Multivariable Analysis: A Practical Guide for Clinicians. Cambridge University Press, Cambridge, UK.

Sackett, D.L., et al., 2001. Evidence-Based Medicine: How to Practice and Teach EBM, second ed. Churchill Livingstone, Edinburgh, UK.

Step-by-Step Biostatistics of a Clinical Trial

The objective of Part III is to present the essentials of biostatistics applied in an intervention clinical study (randomized clinical trial) in a step-by-step manner. For optimal assimilation, the reader should study the steps sequentially.

Chapter 4

Step 1: Investigator's Hypothesis and Expression of its Corresponding Outcome

Every scientific investigation starts with an investigator who (1) observes a phenomenon; (2) raises a question regarding some aspect of this phenomenon; (3) formulates a hypothesis based on this question, either to explain the phenomenon or to establish some kind of correlation; (4) tests his or her hypothesis under controlled conditions; and (5) expresses his or her conclusion.

Although the previous methodology applies to every scientific project conceived in any field, some differences in interpreting study results and applying learned principles prevail among the various disciplines. For example, the study object in medical sciences does not behave in a deterministic manner, as it does in exact sciences. For instance, we could not insert biological data from a patient into a mathematical formula in order to predict with 100% certainty if he or she might respond to a certain medication and if it will be safe for him or her. Therefore, it is necessary to apply tools that will at the least be capable of determining efficacy and safety probabilities regarding a drug, vaccine, or medical procedure.

In biostatistics, clinical impression is replaced by the more objective probabilistic mathematics, in which counted observations in a population are analyzed through statistical models suitable to the investigator's hypothesis and to study type and design. Nevertheless, different from the practice setting, in which we may state that a diagnosis is likely or a given therapy is prone to work, in the probabilistic setting, we must assume that any given correlation is a casual finding (null hypothesis, H_0) and that this casuality must be "pushed aside" until a minimum probabilistic value (generally 5%) is reached in order to accept that whatever was concluded is not casual (alternative hypothesis, H_1). For instance, we conclude that there is an association between propranolol and decreased blood pressure, expressing it as follows: There is a 95% probability that this conclusion is not casual (H_1) and a 5% probability that it is casual (H_0). An H_1 of 95% is generally accepted as sufficient to "push H_0 aside" (or, in more practical terms, to

M. Suchmacher & M. Geller: Practical Biostatistics. DOI: 10.1016/B978-0-12-415794-1.00004-5

TABLE 4.1 The Four Possible Situations in Hypothesis Testing

		Absolute Truth	
		+	−
Your Finding	+	Situation A	Situation B
	−	Situation C	Situation D

reject it). From a clinical standpoint, this would be sufficient to take the finding that propranolol lowers blood pressure as a scientific fact.

All the above means that there is not 100% absolute certainty in biostatistics and in evidence-based medicine but only a 5% probability that one is incorrect (and, consequently, a 95% probability that one is correct). In other words, the aim of most clinical research is to try to reject H_0 and to express its conclusions correspondingly.

In order to further detail this type of approach, consider a table that crosses the findings of your study with absolute truth (Table 4.1).

- Situation A: The association you found coincides with the absolute truth; that is, it is not casual.
- Situation B: The association you found does not coincide with the absolute truth; that is, it is casual. This is a type I error (tolerance for this type of error is conventionally 5%).
- Situation C: You conclude that the association you found is casual when in fact it is not. This is a type II error (tolerance for this type of error is conventionally 20%).
- Situation D: You conclude that the association you found is casual, and that coincides with truth.

Normally, situation A is the one pursued in clinical research; that is, we wish to demonstrate that a medication or a vaccine works, not the opposite. Therefore, we can express a conclusion by stating that p (type I error probability) inferred from a study is less than, equal to, or greater than α (statistical significance level that corresponds to the highest tolerable cutoff for type I error − often 5%, or 0.05), as pre-established by the investigator. Thus, p (or p_α) $< \alpha$ would authorize us to reject H_0 and to accept H_1. An example of the previous proposition can be expressed as follows:

We concluded that the combination trimethoprim−sulfamethoxazole was effective for Pneumocystis jirovecii *lung infection in the HIV-carrier sample studied (*p < 0.05).

This statement can be interpreted as follows: There is a less than a 5% probability that the conclusion represents an error − that is, that the association between *Pneumocystis jirovecii* lung infection cure in the HIV-carrier sample studied and trimethoprim—sulfamethoxazole is a coincidence.

Therefore, it is evident that the goal of clinical research is most often to determine if $p < \alpha$. Many mathematical tools are available to establish these correlations, and from these one is chosen by the biostatistician and the investigator as the most appropriate for the planned study design. Selecting them is a process involving many different elements and stages, which are detailed in the following chapters.

In addition, from a medical perspective, a type II error is as concerning as a type I error. Therefore, why is tolerance for a type II error higher than that for a type I error? The answer is that in practice, it is more difficult to confirm a null hypothesis than an alternative hypothesis. For example, it more difficult to confirm that a patient does not have cancer (we find no signs whatsoever but, perhaps, the disease is so incipient that the a clinical diagnosis is impossible) than to confirm that he or she does have cancer (conspicuous clinical picture of weight loss, tumoral mass, and histopathological findings). (One consequence of this assumption is depicted in Chapter 5.)

Step 2: *n* Estimation and *n* Assessment of a Published Trial

One of the most sensitive tasks in biostatistics is to determine *n* or sample size. This is so because, ideally, a clinical trial should include the totality of individuals in the world carrying the specific condition considered in order to apply its results with the highest possible level of certainty. This would obviously be impossible. Therefore, a convenient resource is sampling from a population based on an assumed ideal *n*, with the aim of further extrapolating biostatistical test results back to this population with a reasonable degree of safety.

Although there is no "correct" or "incorrect" *n*, the sampling process should ensure that the sample is minimally representative of the original population. In order to achieve this goal, sampling should ideally adhere to the guidelines discussed in this chapter.

5.1 FACTORS INFLUENCING *n* DETERMINATION

Two types of factors that influence *n* determination – empirical factors and mathematical factors – must be taken into account before proceeding with its calculation.

5.1.1 Empirical Factors

Empirical factors correspond to subjective and logistic considerations weighted by the investigator and the biostatistician, and they are imprecise in nature. The following factors are usually considered:

- Historical data from previous studies
- Data from pilot studies in cases in which there are no historical data
- Data derived from experimental models
- Effect size, which may represent a relevant difference from a clinical standpoint
- Biological characteristics of the studied condition

M. Suchmacher & M. Geller: Practical Biostatistics. DOI: 10.1016/B978-0-12-415794-1.00005-7
47

- Feasible recruiting rate in the research center(s)
- Study type (e.g. crossover studies probably demand a smaller n for reasons discussed in Chapter 1)
- Eligibility criteria (narrow eligibility criteria lead to a more homogenous population, probably affording a smaller n)
- Condition prevalence and frequency of corresponding complications
- Time available for study completion

5.1.2 Mathematical Factors

Mathematical factors afford a more precise approach to n determination, even though it will still be an approximation.

Statistical Power of the Test

Statistical power of the test corresponds to the capacity of a given statistical test (step 6; see Chapter 9) to effectively find a difference between two compared groups — in other words, the capacity of rejecting H_0 (null hypothesis) when it is false. If it is not sufficiently powerful, existing differences might not be detected, making the investigator incur a type II error. Obviously, the smaller the odds a detected difference should represent an error, the greater the odds this difference actually exists. As such, this power can be expressed in a probabilistic format by the following formula:

$$\text{Statistical power of the test} = 1 - \beta$$

where β represents the statistical significance level that corresponds to the highest degree of tolerability for a statistical test in not detecting a difference — that is, 0.20 (an alternative way of expressing this information is that the tolerance for type II error is 20%). Thus, statistical power of the test can be calculated as follows:

$$\text{Statistical power of the test} = 1 - 0.20 = 0.80 \text{ (or 80\%)}$$

Therefore, 80% would be the lowest acceptable degree of probability of a given statistical test in finding a difference between the groups of a study. Elevating n could by itself increase this probability. In summary, the higher n, the higher the probability of a statistical test finding a difference between groups and, by inference, its power.

Could we make our test statistically more "powerful" by decreasing β to the same value as α (0.05)? Yes, but if we did so, the statistical power of the test would increase up to 0.95 (or 95%), considerably increasing the difficulty in rejecting the null hypothesis (Step 1; see Chapter 4). This would push n to such high figures that it would probably make most clinical trials unviable.

Effect Size

Effect size corresponds to the difference between the results of two groups. For example, a sample of female patients with hyperthyroidism is divided into two groups, with free serum thyroxin levels as the study endpoint, measured at the end of the trial: group A, treated with a test antithyroid drug (2.1 ng/dL), and group B, treated with a reference drug (22.0 ng/dL). Effect size is 19.9 ng/dL.

Some effect size associated factors can influence its impact on *n* determination.

Effect Size Magnitude

Effect size magnitude corresponds to the magnitude (or size) of yielded difference between the results of two groups. Depending on the condition studied and the trial goals, an adequate *n* will be necessary in order to yield a clinically significant effect size between study groups. As a general rule, the smaller the effect size magnitude expected to yield a clinically significant difference, the larger *n* must be, and vice versa. If effect size does not correspond to a sufficient magnitude to yield a clinically significant difference and a small *n* is adopted, the likelihood for type II error is expected to be higher.

Dispersal Degree of Study Results

If yielded results are excessively dispersed, it can become difficult to detect differences between results of different groups. For example, troponin T serum levels (ng/mL) from a group of five subjects with myocardial infarction treated with thrombolytics 1 h after onset of symptoms (group A) are compared with the results from another group of five patients with the same diagnosis treated 4 h after onset of symptoms (group B) (Figure 5.1).

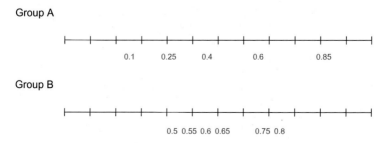

FIGURE 5.1   Schematic representation of the results of troponin T serum levels from group A and group B.

Notice from Figure 5.1 how group A results are more dispersed in comparison to group B results. In such circumstances, it would become difficult to assign the detected difference between groups to either the early administration of thrombolytics or to a casual variability of results. Test power would therefore be diminished. Increasing n could compensate for this limitation by diluting this variability.

Test Direction

Test direction refers to the types of answers an investigator's hypothesis allows. Test direction can be of two types:

- One-sided: Only one type of result direction is possible. For example, could surgical antibiotic prophylaxis decrease postsurgical infection incidence?
- Two-sided: Two opposing answers are possible. For example, what would be the effect of surgical antibiotic prophylaxis on postsurgical infection incidence (would it increase or decrease it)? Bilateral studies demand a higher n in order to make an effect size attainable.

p

The smaller the assumed cutoff for p (generally 0.05), the higher n must be.

Refusals and Dropouts

One must always take refusals and dropouts into account during n determination for a trial. The corresponding n' can be determined by the following formula:

$$n' = \frac{n}{(1 - q)}$$

where $n' = n$ after taking refusals and dropouts into account, and q is the expected proportion of refusals and dropouts.

For example, during study planning, an n of 65 is estimated, and a proportion of 10% of refusals and dropouts is expected:

$$n' = \frac{65}{(1 - 0.10)} = 72$$

n should be 72 so that the study finishes with 65 subjects.

5.2 *n* CALCULATION

The methods discussed in this section are applicable for equal-sized groups.

5.2.1 For Studies Aiming to Analyze Differences Between Means

Calculation of n is performed in two steps.

Standardized Difference Determination

Comparing two different effect sizes requires considering them in the context of the intrinsic variability of the studied endpoint. For example, a 20 IU/L mean decrease in aspartate aminotransferase (AST) serum levels in a context of a standard deviation (step 4; see Chapter 7) of ±30 IU/L is more significant than a 20 IU/L mean decrease in a context of a standard deviation of ±60 IU/L (a wider standard deviation points to the existence of higher discrete (i.e. individual, single) serum AST measurements).

Standardized difference is an index that affords an estimate of the relevance of this difference. It combines the target difference − the minimal effect size considered as clinically relevant expected to be found in the upcoming trial − and the established standard deviation for the studied endpoint. Obviously, standard deviation cannot be known in advance of study performance. Therefore, it must be determined through historical data from similar studies or from pilot studies, or it must be based on empirical clinical grounds.

Standardized difference is calculated by the following formula:

$$\text{Standardized difference} = \frac{\text{target difference}}{\text{standard deviation}}$$

For example, we want to determine the standardized difference for a test anti-hypertensive drug, considering a blood pressure of 15 mmHg as the target difference in a ±25 mmHg standard deviation context:

$$\text{Standardized difference} = \frac{15}{25} = 0.6$$

n Determination

By Applying a Sample Size Nomogram

Test power, standardized difference, and the chosen significance level are applied to a sample size nomogram. By applying the previously discussed example (Figure 5.2):

- Test power = 80% (or 0.80)
- Standardized difference = 0.6
- $p = 0.05$

n would be approximately 80 (40 individuals to each group).

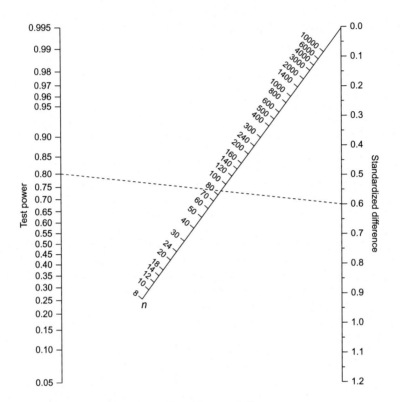

FIGURE 5.2   Sample size nomogram adjusted for $p < 0.05$.

By Applying a Sample Size Formula for Calculation of n of an Individual Group

$$n_i = \frac{2}{d^2} \cdot C_{p,\text{power}}$$

where n_i is the n of an individual group, d is the standardized difference, and $C_{p,\text{power}}$ is the constant defined by p and test power.

$C_{p,\text{power}}$ can be determined according to Table 5.1.

$$n_i = \frac{2}{0.6^2} \cdot 7.9 = 44$$

n_i would be 44 (therefore, n would be 88).

Note that sample size nomogram and sample size formula do not necessarily have to yield the exact same values because their objective is to give n estimates.

TABLE 5.1 Constant *p* Versus Power Determination

p	Test Power			
	50	*80*	*90*	*95*
0.05	3.8	7.9	10.5	13.0

5.2.2 For Studies Aiming to Analyze Differences Between Proportions

For example, based on historical and empirical data, we infer that the expected 1-year survival rate for pleural mesothelioma treated with a cisplatin plus gemcitabine regimen is 42% compared to a 32% survival rate with an oxaliplatin plus raltitrexed regimen. We want to estimate *n* in order to develop a formal study on this issue comparing group A (cisplatin plus gemcitabine) with group B (oxaliplatin plus raltitrexed).

Calculation of *n* is performed in two steps.

Standardized Difference Determination

Standardized difference determination is calculated by the following formula:

$$\text{Standardized difference} = \frac{p_A - p_B}{\sqrt{p'(1 - p')}}$$

where p_A is the group A proportion, p_B is the group B proportion, and p' is the arithmetic mean of p_A and p_B:

$$\text{Standardized difference} = \frac{0.42 - 0.32}{\sqrt{0.37(1 - 0.37)}} = 0.2$$

n *Determination*

By Applying a Sample Size Nomogram

Test power, standardized difference, and the chosen significance level are applied to a sample size nomogram. By applying the previously discussed example (Figure 5.3),

- Test power = 80% (or 0.80)
- Standardized difference = 0.20
- *p* = 0.05

n would be 800 (400 subjects to each group).

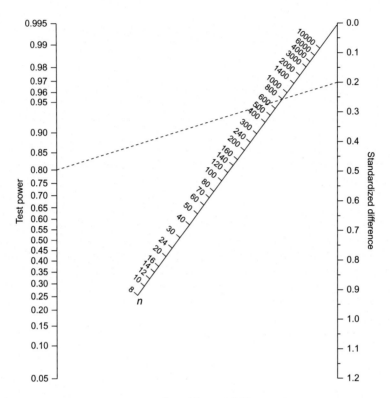

FIGURE 5.3   Sample size nomogram adjusted for $p < 0.05$.

By Applying a Sample Size Formula for Calculation of n of an Individual Group

$$n_i = \frac{[p_A (1 - p_A) + p_B (1 - p_B)]}{(p_A - p_B)^2} \cdot C_{p,power}$$

where n_i is the n of an individual group, p_A is the group A proportion, p_B is the group B proportion, and $C_{p,power}$ is the constant defined by p and test power.

$C_{p,power}$ can be determined according to Table 5.1:

$$n_i = \frac{[0.42 (1 - 0.42) + 0.32 (1 - 0.32)]}{(0.42 - 0.32)^2} \cdot 7.9 = 356$$

n_i would be 356 (therefore, n would be 712).

Note that sample size nomogram and sample size formula do not necessarily have to yield the exact same values because their objective is to give *n* estimates.

The previous examplified values do not represent an absolutely dependable *n* for reaching trustworthy results in clinical trials but, rather, only an approximation. For example, if an *n* of 90 is calculated, it is permissible to rule out the need for an *n* of 600 but not for an *n* of 100. Round ups are also allowed, for instance, from a calculated *n* of 178 to an *n* of 180.

5.3 ASSESSING *n* OF A PUBLISHED TRIAL

The methods discussed in this section are applicable for equal-sized groups.

By estimating the respective test power, it is possible to indirectly estimate whether *n* of a published trial was adequate to attain the objective of a study.

In order to determine *n*, we first had to choose the significance level and test power and then find the standardized difference. Now, for determining test power, we must first find the standardized difference — according to published study results — and then apply it, the significance level, and *n* chosen in the published trial to the sample size nomogram.

5.3.1 Studies that Analyzed Differences Between Means

For example, in a study with an *n* of 200 subjects with chronic obstructive pulmonary disease (COPD), 95 patients were randomized to group A (bronchodilators + nasal O_2) and 105 to group B (only bronchodilators) in order to compare arterial pO_2 with each modality. Chosen significance level was 0.05. Mean arterial pO_2 in group A was 95 mmHg, and mean arterial pO_2 in group B was 93 mmHg (i.e. a 2 mmHg difference). According to literature data, the standard deviation for arterial pO_2 in COPD patients treated only with bronchodilators is ±5 mmHg. Standardized difference is determined by the same formula as that presented previously:

$$\text{Standardized difference} = \frac{\text{target difference}}{\text{standard deviation}} = \frac{2}{5} = 0.4$$

By applying data to the sample size nomogram, we obtain Figure 5.4.

We can verify that the test power applied in this published trial was 0.80, and that in order to find such a 2 mmHg difference under a test power or 0.80, an *n* of approximately 200 would have been necessary.

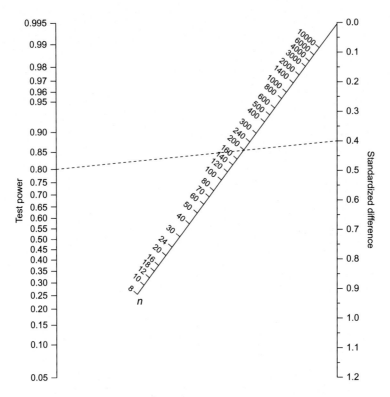

FIGURE 5.4   Sample size nomogram adjusted for $p < 0.05$.

5.3.2 Studies that Analyzed Differences Between Proportions

For example, in a study with an n of 390 subjects with moderate bilateral knee osteoarthritis, 189 patients were randomized to group A (physical therapy) and 201 to group B (an OA modifying drug) in order to compare pain improvement with each modality. Chosen significance level was 0.05. Thirty-eight percent of subjects presented pain improvement in group A compared to 29% in group B (i.e. a 9% difference). Standardized difference is calculated by the same formula as that presented previously:

$$\text{Standardized difference} = \frac{p_A - p_B}{\sqrt{p'(1-p')}} = \frac{0.38 - 0.29}{\sqrt{0.33(1-0.33)}} = 0.20$$

By applying data to the sample size nomogram, we obtain Figure 5.5.

We can verify that test power applied in this published trial would have been approximately 0.55 (continuous line), and that for finding such a 9% difference under a test power or 0.80, an n of approximately 650 would have been necessary (Figure 5.5, dotted line).

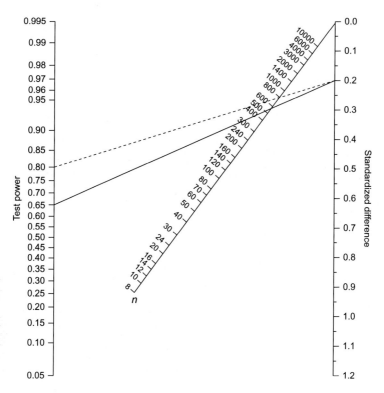

FIGURE 5.5   Sample size nomogram adjusted for $p < 0.05$.

Chapter 6

Step 3: Organization of Variables and Endpoints

The term "variable" refers to any parameter that varies and can be measured (e.g. potassium serum levels, height, and QRS complex amplitude). Endpoints are the predictive variables (or efficacy variables) chosen as the comparison parameters meant to determine the outcome between the groups of a clinical trial. Both determine the biostatistical model to be adopted. They can be classified as qualitative variables and quantitative variables.

6.1 QUALITATIVE VARIABLES

Qualitative variables do not allow for the direct assignment of absolute numerical values. An assigned value cannot, in principle, be greater or smaller than the other.

6.1.1 Categorical

Categorical (nominal) variables express characteristics rather than numerical values, and they do not allow for ordering (e.g. eye color and type of pain sensation). Nevertheless, in order to make statistical testing possible, the biostatistician eventually needs to assign them numerical values through appropriate tools:

- Dichotomous variables: Dichotomous variables admit two mutually exclusive categories (e.g. yes or no, male or female, and life or death).
- Nondichotomous variables: Nondichotomous variables admit two or more non-mutually exclusive categories (e.g. simple, cominutive, or open fracture; and short, moderate, or prolonged sun exposure).

6.1.2 Ordinal

In the ordinal variables setting, ordering is admissible, although interval sizes between orders are not quantifiable (e.g. edema intensity (mild, moderate, or severe) and social level (high, average, or low)). Alternatively, categories can be replaced by ranks in order to facilitate hypothesis testing (Step 6; Chapter 9).

M. Suchmacher & M. Geller: Practical Biostatistics. DOI: 10.1016/B978-0-12-415794-1.00006-9

One should be aware that biostatistical test results and interpretation will inevitably bear some imprecision because the initial categorization is elaborated on a subjective basis.

6.2 QUANTITATIVE VARIABLES

In the quantitative variables setting, values are numerically collected and expressed, and intervals between these values are equal (e.g. intracranial pressure, body temperature, and number of cells/mm^3).

6.2.1 Discrete

In the discrete (i.e. individual, single) variables setting, only whole values are admissible (e.g. number of pregnancies or convulsion episodes). They are used basically for counting events. Discrete variables are generally associated with event counting.

6.2.2 Continuous

Continuous (interval) variables refer to whole values and their fractions (e.g. age (1 year and 3 months) and body weight (48.2 kg)). Continuous variables are generally associated with some measurement procedure.

After collection, variable values are tabulated according to study design. Clinical research tables are structured as rows, columns, blocks, and repetitions (observations) that correspond to individual subjects. An example is shown in Table 6.1.

Tabulation is the first step in defining the distribution pattern of collected variables: normal or non-normal (Step 5; Chapter 8). This is a defining issue regarding the selection of one of the two main biostatistical test groups to be applied: parametric (involves normal distribution) or nonparametric (does not involve normal distribution). The best statistical test to determine if $p < \alpha$ will be selected based on this choice.

TABLE 6.1 Placebo-Controlled Efficacy Study on an Oral Hypoglycemic Drug

Treated Group	Tested Medication					
	Fasting serum glucose (mg/dL)					
	Oral hypoglycemic drug			Placebo		
Therapeutic group						
Subject 1	102	101	98	134	130	221
Subject 2	95	122	130	131	128	150
Subject 3	109	115	191	409	199	199
Subject 4	99	100	110	97	333	161
Subject 5	77	101	100	102	155	320
Placebo group						
Subject 1	99	100	110	131	128	150
Subject 2	102	101	98	102	155	320
Subject 3	77	101	100	97	333	161
Subject 4	95	122	130	409	199	199
Subject 5	109	115	191	134	130	221

Chapter 7

Step 4: Measures for Results Expression of a Clinical Trial

As previously discussed, data frequency distribution from a study can be tabulated. However, because it is not practical to express study results in this manner, specific summarizing measures are usually adopted. In normal data distribution studies (Step 5; Chapter 8), those data tend to concentrate around a mean and then to disperse bidirectionally. Hence, in this setting, we can propose two main types of summarizing parameters: central tendency and dispersal measures. In addition to summarizing study data, both are useful in estimating biological qualities of the enrolled sample.

By convention, the symbols used to express some of the central tendency and dispersal measures are expressed in Greek and English characters for populations and samples, respectively: (1) μ (pronounced as "mu"), mean for population; (2) σ (sigma), standard deviation for population; (3) $\bar{x}$ (pronounced as "x bar"), for samples; and (4) S, standard deviation for samples.

7.1 CENTRAL TENDENCY MEASURES

Central tendency measures used are mean, median and mode.

7.1.1 Mean

Mean (arithmetic mean) ($\bar{x}$ or μ) is the measure that best represents the centrality of a population or sample. This proximity is directly proportional to the following parameters: (1) N or n, respectively; (2) homogeneity of data distribution; and (3) number of observations. It is a useful measure for continuous variables. For example, the results of serum total cholesterol measurements from a 10-patient sample are detailed in Table 7.1 for mean determination.

The formula for mean calculation is

$$\bar{x} = \frac{\sum x_i}{n}$$

M. Suchmacher & M. Geller: Practical Biostatistics. DOI: 10.1016/B978-0-12-415794-1.00007-0

TABLE 7.1 Results of Serum Total Cholesterol Levels in a Sample of 10 Patients

Patient No.	Serum Total Cholesterol (mg/dL)
Patient 1	241
Patient 2	190
Patient 3	202
Patient 4	210
Patient 5	299
Patient 6	256
Patient 7	249
Patient 8	184
Patient 9	213
Patient 10	236

where $\sum$ is summation, x_i is the individual variable result, and n is the number of individuals.

$$\bar{x} = \frac{241 + 190 + 202 + 210 + 299 + 256 + 249 + 184 + 213 + 236}{10}$$
$$= 228 \text{ mg/dL}$$

A limitation of mean is that outliers can significantly deviate it from the value that summarizes the sample or population. Consider a second example based on the same sample, in which two outliers replace the values of patients 1 and 6 (Table 7.2).

7.1.2 Median

If the values of a variable from a population or sample are disposed in a crescent manner, then median corresponds to the value from which half the values are above it and the other half below it. For example, a sample of 11 infants with a diagnosis of *Haemophilus influenzae* meningitis was submitted to lumbar puncture for white cell count in cerebrospinal fluid (Table 7.3). White cell count results are displayed in a crescent manner in Figure 7.1.

TABLE 7.2 Results of Serum Total Cholesterol Levels with Two Outliers (In Bold)

Patient No.	Total Serum Cholesterol (mg/dL)
Patient 1	**110**
Patient 2	190
Patient 3	202
Patient 4	210
Patient 5	299
Patient 6	**492**
Patient 7	249
Patient 8	184
Patient 9	213
Patient 10	236

TABLE 7.3 Results of White Cell Count in Cerebrospinal Fluid in an 11-Infants Sample

Patient No.	White Cell Count (mm^3)
Patient 1	4600
Patient 2	4000
Patient 3	4600
Patient 4	3500
Patient 5	5000
Patient 6	4250
Patient 7	4550
Patient 8	4500
Patient 9	5500
Patient 10	3600
Patient 11	4200

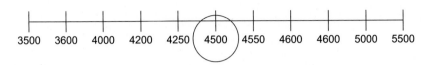

FIGURE 7.1　Schematic representation of the ordering of Table 7.3 white cell counts.

Median is 4500 because there are five values above it and five below. Differently from mean, median is relatively protected against outliers. For example, if the value from patient 9 was 100,000 instead of 5500 white cells/mm^3, median would still remain 4500. For similar reasons, median is especially useful for observations with an asymmetrical distribution. A small possibility for mathematical manipulation is its limitation. For samples with an even number of individuals, median will correspond to the mean of the two central values.

7.1.3 Mode

Mode corresponds to the value with the largest number of observations in a population or sample. In the example discussed in Section 7.1.2, mode would be 4600. Because there may be more than one most frequently observed value, there may be more than one mode. Correspondingly, if there are no values with two or more repetitions, there will be no mode. It is a useful measure for qualitative values. Mode is a position measure rather than a central tendency measure, given the fact that it indicates the point where the largest number of observations is concentrated, which is not necessarily centrally located.

7.2 DISPERSAL MEASURES

Dispersal measures are amplitude, variance and standard deviation, coefficient of variation, and standard error of the mean.

7.2.1 Amplitude

Amplitude corresponds to the difference between the largest and smallest value in a population or sample. In the example in Section 7.1.1 (Table 7.1), the amplitude would be 114 mg/dL. Amplitude does not provide information regarding data dispersal or robustness against outliers.

7.2.2 Variance and Standard Deviation

As observed in Section 7.1.1, the more dispersed the data from a population or sample, the smaller the homogeneity expected from this population or sample, from a biological standpoint. One way of measuring this dispersivity is to calculate its mean and then to determine the difference (deviation) between each one of its data points and the mean. Let us check the example of Section 7.1.1 again (Table 7.1). Its mean is 228, and deviations are detailed in Table 7.4.

Notwithstanding, to obtain only the deviations of a sample would not suffice to measure its degree of dispersal. In order to infer it, one must determine the variance (σ^2 for populations and S^2 for samples), which is a measure that condenses all individual deviations in such a way that either adding or subtracting it from the mean would provide the range inside which most of the data would tend to concentrate and outside of which the remaining data would tend to disperse. Variance is determined by the following formulas for population and samples respectively:

$$\sigma^2 = \frac{\sum(x_i - \bar{x})^2}{N}$$

$$S^2 = \frac{\sum(x_i - \bar{x})^2}{n - 1}$$

where x_i is the individual variable result, $\bar{x}$ is the mean, and N and n are the number of individuals.

TABLE 7.4 Results of Deviations from the Mean of Table 7.1

Patient No.	Deviation
Patient 1	$241 - 228 = 13$
Patient 2	$190 - 228 = -38$
Patient 3	$202 - 228 = -26$
Patient 4	$210 - 228 = -18$
Patient 5	$299 - 228 = 71$
Patient 6	$256 - 228 = 28$
Patient 7	$249 - 228 = 21$
Patient 8	$184 - 228 = -44$
Patient 9	$213 - 228 = -15$
Patient 10	$236 - 228 = 8$

The deviations are squared because otherwise their sum would equal zero due to the mutual compensation between positive and negative deviations (Table 7.4; $13 + (-38) + (-26) + (-18) + 71 + 28 + 21 + (-44) + (-15) + 8 = 0$). A numerator equal to zero would obviously make the previous equations unviable. By squaring the deviations, they are all turned into positive values, allowing calculation. However, squaring the deviations creates a new unit (mg/dL^2) different from the original one (mg/dL), generating interpretation incongruences. Notwithstanding, this can be corrected by calculating standard deviation ("standard" meaning representative) through the following respective formulas:

$$\sigma = \sqrt{\sigma^2}$$
$$S = \sqrt{S^2}$$

Hence, standard deviation is simply the square root of the variance. Let us use the former example for calculating both:

$$S^2 = \frac{(13)^2 + (-38)^2 + (-26)^2 + (-18)^2 + (71)^2 + (28)^2 + (21)^2 + (-44)^2 + (-15)^2 + (8)^2}{10 - 1}$$

$$= 1233 \, mg/dL^2$$
$$S = \sqrt{1233} = 35 \, mg/dL$$

Thirty-five is subtracted from 228 ($228 - 35 = 193$) and added to it ($228 + 35 = 263$). We can infer that the dispersivity of this sample is represented by the interval 193–263, and that most of its data must be concentrated inside it. An alternative way to express it is 228 ± 35.[1]

The concept of standard deviation may also be schematically represented. Observe the scale in Figure 7.2, and notice the tendency of individual values toward the mean (superior line represents standard deviation range).

Classifying the dispersivity expressed by a standard deviation as narrow or large might depend either on the investigator's interpretation or on the coefficient of variation (see Section 7.2.3). As a general rule, the narrower the standard deviation, the more homogeneous its corresponding population or sample is expected to be.[2]

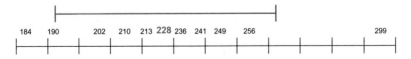

FIGURE 7.2   Schematic representation of a standard deviation from the mean.

---

[1] From a strict algebraic perspective, variance and standard deviation can only be expressed as positive values; nevertheless, for didactic purposes, we also express them as negative values.
[2] Error meaning deviation.

7.2.3 Coefficient of Variation

Standard deviation by itself does not inform on the relative magnitude of the data of a population or sample. For example, a standard deviation of ± 2 has different meanings in a sample of 10 and in a sample of 100 individuals. Therefore, in order to make inferences regarding its relative significance, it is necessary to quantify it for population and sample as a percentual representation of dispersal — the coefficient of variation (CV) — through respective formulas:

$$CV = \frac{\sigma}{\bar{x}} \times 100\%$$

$$CV = \frac{S}{\bar{x}} \times 100\%$$

where σ is the standard deviation (population), S is the standard deviation (sample), and $\bar{x}$ is the mean.

By convention, the following CV values are adopted:

- $<15\%$, low dispersal
- $15 < CV < 30\%$, average dispersal
- $>30\%$, high dispersal

CV affords three types of analysis:

- Dispersal estimate of a population or sample
  - For example, in a sample of patients with chronic persistent hepatitis, we learn that mean total serum bilirubin level is 16 mg/dL and standard deviation ± 3 mg/dL. Because 3 is 19% of 16, CV is 19%.
- Comparative dispersal between different samples
  - For example, in a sample of patients with chronic persistent hepatitis, we learn that mean total serum bilirubin level is 16 mg/dL and standard deviation ± 3 mg/dL; therefore, CV is 19%. In another sample with the same condition, mean total serum bilirubin level is also 16 mg/dL and standard deviation ± 5 mg/dL; therefore, CV is 31%. Thus, although both samples present the same mean, their CVs suggest that they are not biologically homogeneous.
- Comparative dispersal of variables of different nature in the same sample
  - For example, in the same sample, there are overweight individuals presenting a clinical picture of peripheral insulin resistance, mean body weight of 90 ± 15 kg, and mean fasting serum insulin level of 82 ± 19 mg/dL. Body weight and fasting serum insulin level CVs are 16 and 21%, respectively. We notice that CVs of both variables are different, which suggests that this sample is more homogeneous for body weight than for fasting serum insulin level.

7.2.4 Standard Error of the Mean

Previously, we studied mean and standard deviation of a sample and the significance of both. However, we must also take into account that the studied sample has been extracted from a general population, and that these statistics may also present some variability relative to the mean and standard deviation of the general population and remainder samples (Figure 7.3).

In fact, these samples share similar characteristics because they are originated from the same source. On the other hand, they may present different central tendency and dispersal measures among themselves due to n variability and randomness. Therefore, it is necessary to determine their error[2] (i.e. how much their standard deviations are "bent" by their n) before making comparative inferences between central tendency and dispersal measures of two samples and those of the general population and other samples. This is attainable through a dispersal measure termed standard error of the mean, which is calculated by the following formulas for populations and samples, respectively:

$$\sigma_\mu = \frac{\sigma}{\sqrt{N}}$$

where σ is the population standard deviation, and N is the number of individuals in the population.

$$S_{\bar{x}} = \frac{S}{\sqrt{n}}$$

where S is the sample standard deviation, and n is the number of individuals per sample.

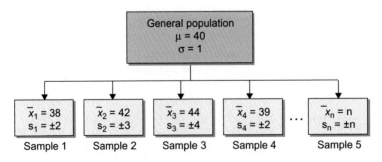

FIGURE 7.3   Schematic representation of a sampling distribution (Step 7; Chapter 10) showing the relationship among general population and samples, with exemplifying statistics.

TABLE 7.5 n and Standard Deviations from a Hypothetical General Population and Respective Samples

	N/n	σ/S
General population	150	3
Sample 1	50	5
Sample 2	20	2

Observe the example shown in Table 7.5:

$$\text{Sample1 } S_{\bar{x}} = \frac{5}{7} = 0.71$$

$$\text{Sample2 } S_{\bar{x}} = \frac{2}{4.4} = 0.45$$

$$\sigma_\mu = \frac{3}{12.2} = 0.24$$

These data indicate that whenever we make comparative inferences, we must take into account that general population standard error of the mean tends to be narrower than that of sample 2, and sample 2 standard error of the mean tends to be narrower than that of sample 1.

7.3 POSITION MEASURES: QUANTILES

Quantiles can be considered as an extension of the concept of median: Whereas the latter divides the sample or population into two equal halves of observations based on a central value, in quantiles more divisions based on equally distanced values are added, forming new ranges with each containing a certain number of observations (but not necessarily the same number of observations). Therefore, quantiles correspond to a form of sample partitioning into equal frequency ranges, generated by measured variables. Quantiles aim (1) to afford a standardized means to position an individual inside a sample, consequently to the corresponding value range; (2) to determine an interval established by extreme positions, which encompasses the majority of these individuals, along with related variable ranges; and (3) to establish an interval of individuals, along with variable ranges determined by two different positions.

By convention, there are 99 partitions generated by 100 centiles. Alternatively, centile 10 (or the 10th percentile) may be named 1st decile, for example, or centile

25 1st quartile (because it corresponds to 1/4 of 100 centiles). The interval between the 25th and 75th percentiles corresponds to the so-called interquartile range, which tends to concentrate most of the individuals of a sample (assuming there is normal distribution (Step 5; Chapter 8)) (Figure 7.4).

Consider the following example: Body mass index (BMI) was determined in a sample of 104 patients. Results are displayed in a frequency distribution table (Table 7.6).

We want to know the following:

- What BMI range contains centile 90 patient (or the 90th percentile)?

  First, we must determine who the patient is (element) who corresponds to the 90th percentile. This can be inferred through a simple rule of three formula:

$$E_c = i \times \frac{n}{100}$$

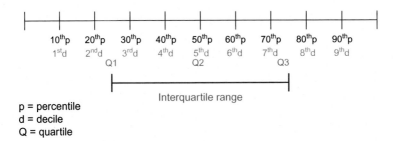

p = percentile
d = decile
Q = quartile

FIGURE 7.4   Schematic representation of an interquartile range.

TABLE 7.6 Frequency Distribution of BMI in a Sample of 104 Patients

BMI (kg/m^2)	r_j	R_j
>16.5	3	3
16.5–18.5	9	12
18.5–25	13	25
25–30	17	42
30–35	25	67
35–40	28	95
>40	9	104

r_j, patients per range; R_j, accumulated patients.

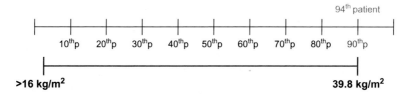

FIGURE 7.5   Schematic representation of the range $>16.5-40$ kg/m^2.

where E_c is the centile element (patient ordinal number), i is the proposed centile, and n is the number of individuals.

$$E_c = 90 \times \frac{104}{100} = 94\text{th element}$$

The R_j column in Table 7.6 shows that the 94th patient belongs to the $35-40$ kg/m^2 BMI range. Therefore, $35-40$ kg/m^2 BMI is the range that contains 90th percentile.

- At what BMI range will a significant proportion of patients (e.g. 90th percentile) be included?

  According to the former inference, this range corresponds to $35-40$ kg/m^2. This could be interpreted in two ways:
  1. 90% of studied patients are included within the >16.5 to 40 kg/m^2 range (Figure 7.5).
  2. An individual with a BMI higher than the $35-40$ kg/m^2 range (95th patient onward) has a BMI greater than 90% of the remaining individuals in the studied sample.

- Inside which BMI range are most of the patients concentrated?

  Because the interquartile range generally includes most of the individuals of a sample, it is expected to correspond to the BMI range inside which most of the patients are concentrated. Therefore, it is necessary to know the patients who correspond to the 25th and 75th percentiles:

$$E_c = i_{25} \times \frac{n}{100} = 26\text{th element}$$

$$E_c = i_{75} \times \frac{n}{100} = 78\text{th element}$$

The BMI table shows that the interquartile range corresponds to the $25-40\ kg/m^2$ range, to which most of the patients belong (Figure 7.6).

One way of expressing these results is a box-and-whiskers plot diagram (with "box" corresponding to the interquartile range and "whiskers" to the whole observations range) (Figure 7.7).

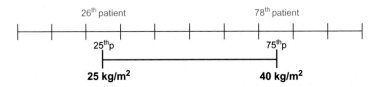

FIGURE 7.6   Schematic representation of the range $25-40\ kg/m^2$.

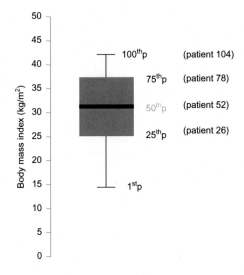

FIGURE 7.7   A box-and-whiskers representation of BMI frequency distribution.

APPENDIX 7.1: HOW TO CALCULATE MEAN USING MICROSOFT EXCEL (SECTION 7.1.1)

Step 1

Tabulate your data, and select the cell immediately inferior to the column of arguments for which you want to calculate the mean (B12). Click on the **Formulas** tag, and then click on the **More Functions** button in the **Function Library** area. Click on the **Statistical** drop-down menu button and then on the **AVERAGE** secondary drop-down menu button for the **Function Arguments** dialog box.

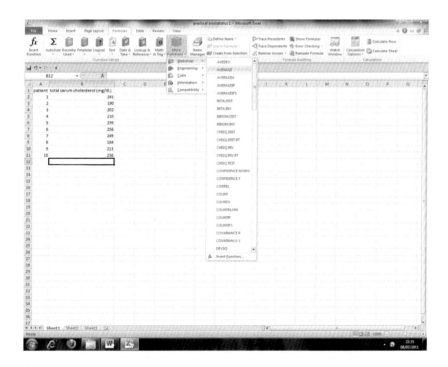

Step 2

AVERAGE formula comprehending B2:B11 array is shown in the B12 cell. B2:B11 array is shown in the **Number 1** field of the **Function Arguments** dialog box. Mean is shown in the result space.

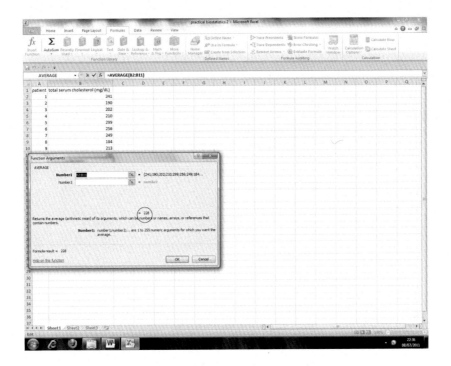

APPENDIX 7.2: HOW TO "TRIM" THE MEAN OF OUTLIERS (SECTION 7.1.1)

To "trim" a mean corresponds to ignoring outliers from its calculation based on a conventional percentage that excludes the highest and the lowest outliers.

Step 1

Tabulate your data and select the cell immediately inferior to the column of arguments whose mean you wish to trim (B12). Click on the **Formulas** tag and then on the **More Functions** button in the **Function Library** area. Click on the **Statistical** drop-down menu button and then on the **TRIMMEAN** secondary drop-down menu button for the **Function Arguments** dialog box.

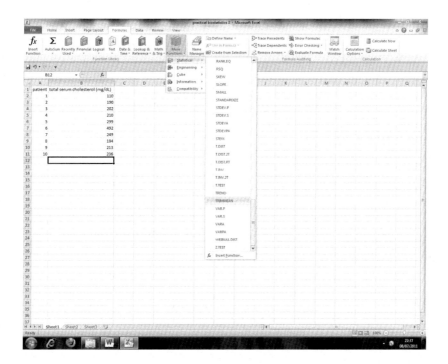

Step 2

TRIMMEAN formula comprehending B2:B11 array is shown in B12 cell. Put your cursor in the **Array** field. Then select the B2:B11 array on the sheet itself. The array is shown in the **Array** field. Then insert the percentage related to the outliers you wish to trim in the **Percent** field; in our example, it is 0.2 (note that you must express percentages as decimals). This percentage trims arguments 110 (B2) and 492 (B7) from the formula. **TRIMMEAN** is shown in the result space.

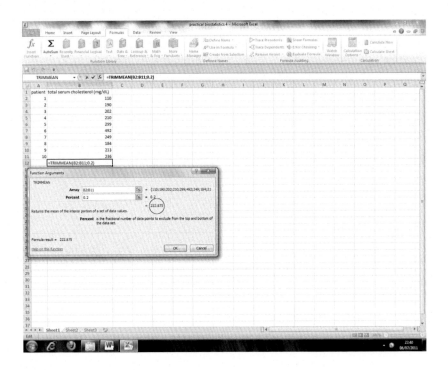

APPENDIX 7.3: HOW TO DETERMINE MEDIAN USING MICROSOFT EXCEL (SECTION 7.1.2)

Step 1

Tabulate your data, and select the cell immediately inferior to the column of arguments for which you want to calculate the median (B13). Click on the **Formulas** tag and then on the **More Functions** button in the **Function Library** area. Click on the **Statistical** drop-down menu button and then on the **MEDIAN** secondary drop-down menu button for the **Function Arguments** dialog box.

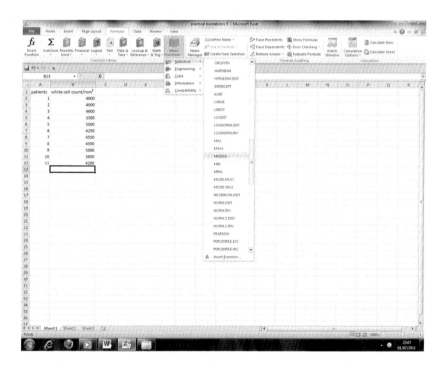

Step 2

MEDIAN formula comprehending B2:B11 array is shown in the B12 cell. Put your cursor in the **Number 1** field. Then select B2:B12 array on the sheet itself. The array is shown in the **Number 1** field. **MEDIAN** is shown in the result space.

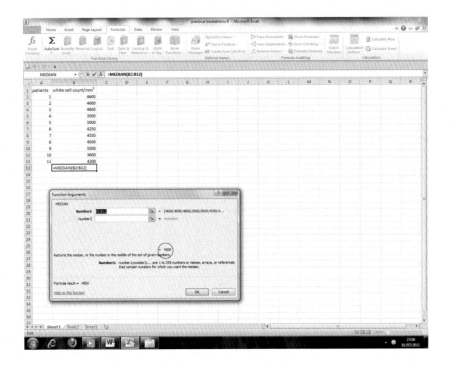

APPENDIX 7.4: HOW TO DETERMINE MODE USING MICROSOFT EXCEL (SECTION 7.1.3)

Step 1

Tabulate your data, and select the cell immediately inferior to the column of arguments for which you want to determine the mode (B13). Click on the **Formulas** tag and then on the **More Functions** button in the **Function Library** area. Click on the **Statistical** drop-down menu button and then on the **MODE.SNGL** (MODE.SiNGLe) secondary drop-down menu button for the **Function Arguments** dialog box.

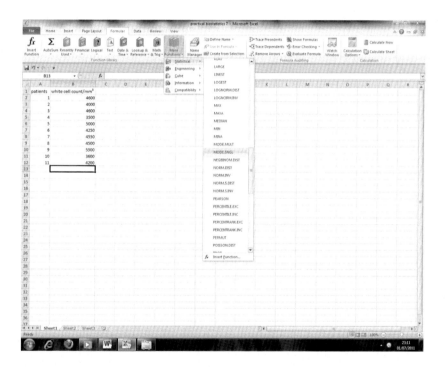

Step 2

Mode formula comprehending B2:B12 array is shown in B13 cell. Put your cursor in the **Number 1** field. Then select B2:B12 array on the sheet itself. The array is shown in the **Number 1** field. Mode is shown in the result space.

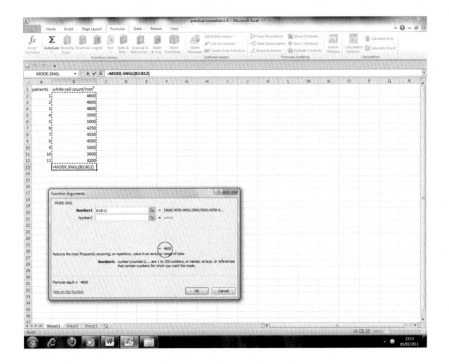

APPENDIX 7.5: HOW TO CALCULATE STANDARD DEVIATION USING MICROSOFT EXCEL (SECTION 7.2.2)

Step 1

Tabulate your data and select the cell immediately inferior to the column of arguments for which you want to calculate standard deviation (B12). Click on the **Formulas** tag and then on the **More Functions** button in the **Function Library** area. Click on the **Statistical** drop-down menu button and then on the **STDEV.S** (STandard DEViation.Sample) secondary drop-down menu button for the **Function Arguments** dialog box.

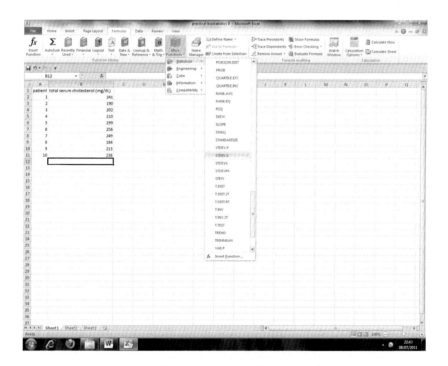

Step 2

Standard deviation formula comprehending B2:B11 array is shown in B12 cell. Put your cursor in the **Number 1** field. Then select B2:B11 array on the sheet itself. The array is shown in the **Number 1** field. Standard deviation is shown in the result space.

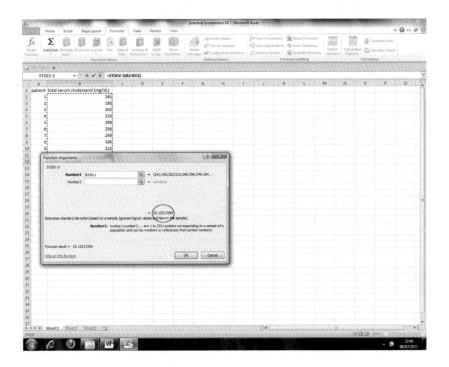

APPENDIX 7.6: HOW TO FIND THE EXACT BMI THAT CORRESPONDS TO THE 90TH PERCENTILE USING MICROSOFT EXCEL (SECTION 7.3)

Step 1

Tabulate your data, and select the cell immediately inferior to the column of arguments for which you want to find the 90th percentile (A:16). Click on the **Formulas** tag and then on the **More Functions** button in the **Function Library** area. Click on the **Statistical** drop-down menu button and then on **the PERCENTILE.INC** secondary drop-down menu button for the **Function Arguments** dialog box.

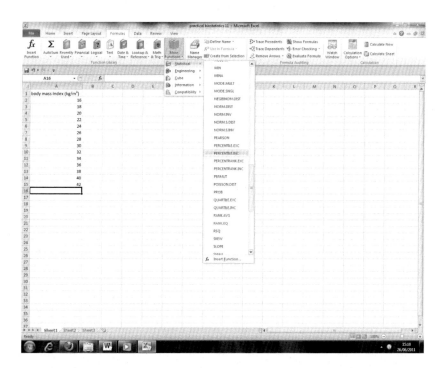

Step 2

Percentile formula comprehending A2:A15 array is shown in A16 cell. Put your cursor in the **Array** field and then select B2:B15 array on the sheet itself. Insert the percentage related to the percentile you want to find in the **K** field, 0.9 (note that you must express percentages as decimals). Percentile is shown in the result space.

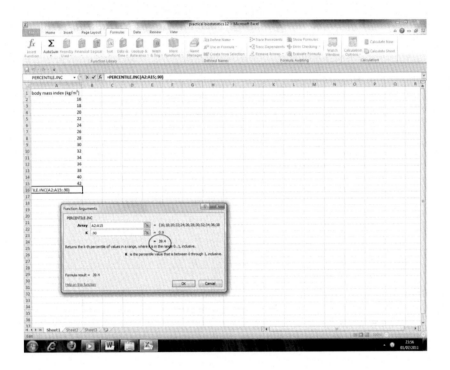

The 90th percentile corresponds to 39.4 kg/m^2 BMI. Therefore, the 90th percentile belongs to the 35–40 kg/m^2 BMI range.

APPENDIX 7.7: HOW TO PUT ALL BMIs IN A "RANK AND PERCENTILE" PERSPECTIVE USING MICROSOFT EXCEL (SECTION 7.3)

Step 1

Tabulate patients (A2:A105) and respective BMIs (B2:B105). Click on the **Data** tag and then on the **Data Analysis** button in the **Analysis** area for the **Data Analysis** dialog box. Select the **Rank and Percentile** option, and click **OK**. A **Rank and Percentile** dialog box opens.

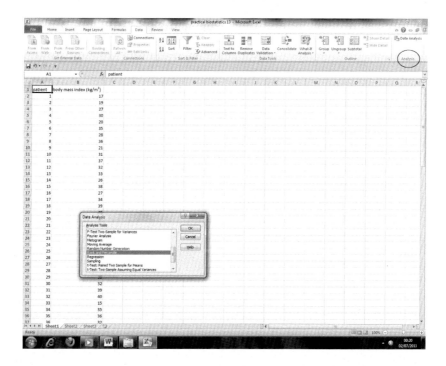

Step 2

Checkmark the **Output Range** circle at **Output options** for you to choose the array in which you want your rank and percentile data to be exhibited. Put your cursor in the **Output Range** field and select the array on the sheet itself (D1:G105). It will be shown in the **Output Range** field. Put your cursor in the **Input Range** field and select the array of the original BMIs data on the sheet itself, disregarding the column's name (B2:B105). Click **OK**.

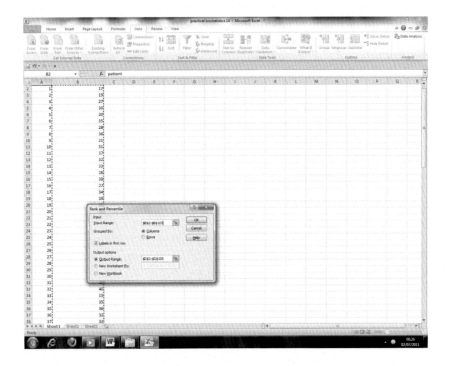

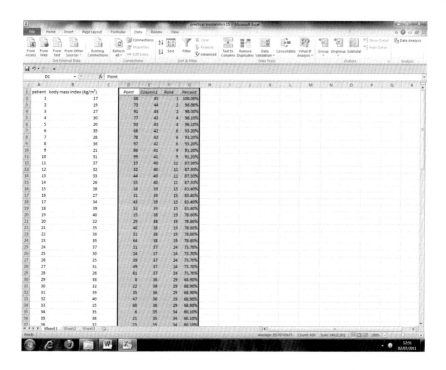

By default, Excel identifies the first column of the new table as **Point** and the second column as **Column1**. You can replace both with the headings of the original table **Patient** and **Body Mass Index (kg/m²)**, respectively.

As can be seen, patient 88 has the 1st rank and corresponds to the 100th percentile, patient 73 has the 2nd rank and corresponds to the 98th percentile, patient 91 has the 3rd rank and corresponds to 98th percentile, and so forth.

Chapter 8

Step 5: Determination of Normality or Non-Normality of Data Distribution

Due to their biological nature, it is expected that values collected from a human population follow a typical distribution pattern characterized by (1) a central mean that represents most of these values and (2) the remaining values, which become less frequent as they move away from this mean. For example, a sample of 100 individuals is studied for mean white blood cell count determination, and the results are shown in Table 8.1.

Notice that the median, 7000 cells/mm^3, concentrates most of the individuals, and that the number of individuals decreases as they move away from it. This type of data distribution is termed normal because data distribution in a "normal" population is considered as such. A graphic representation of the distribution of white blood cell counts from this sample is represented in Figure 8.1.

The type of symmetrical curve generated by a normal distribution, as shown previously, is termed a normal curve. Most of clinical trial data follow a normal distribution pattern because this is the "normal" tendency of biological phenomena.

As shown previously, the normal curve is prone to present a typical bell-shaped form, determined by a mathematical formula (not shown) that includes mean and standard deviation parameters. Therefore, in order to determine if a given distribution pattern is normal or not, a necessary step is to plot study data and to verify their curve shape. For this purpose, tabulated data are transposed to a conventional graphic distribution pattern known as a Gauss curve. This mathematical resource has the following characteristics:

- Gauss curve values, termed Z-scores, correspond to study data expressed as standard deviations (SD) and are determined by a mathematical formula (discussed later).
- Z-scores range from −3 SD to +3 SD and are placed on the the horizontal axis.
- Mean corresponds to a Z-score of 0, with positive SD on the right side and negative SD on the left side.
- Research subjects are placed on the vertical axis.

M. Suchmacher & M. Geller: Practical Biostatistics. DOI: 10.1016/B978-0-12-415794-1.00008-2

TABLE 8.1 Results of White Blood Cell Counts in a Sample of 100 Individuals

	White Blood Cell Counts (Cells/mm³)								
	2000	3000	4000	5000	7000	9000	10000	11000	12000
No. of individuals	2	3	5	15	50	15	5	3	2

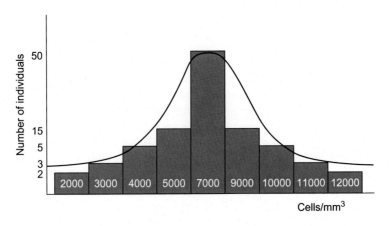

FIGURE 8.1   Graphic distribution of white blood cell counts in a sample of 100 individuals.

The critical ratio formula is used to convert study data into Z-scores:

$$Z = \frac{x - \mu}{\sigma}$$

$$Z = \frac{x - \bar{x}}{S}$$

where x is the variable value, $\mu/\bar{x}$ are the mean (populations and samples, respectively), and σ/S are the standard deviation (populations and samples, respectively).

Gauss curve (Figure 8.2) presents characteristics that make it useful in biostatistics:

- It would not be practical to perform plottings for all possible data and unit types used in clinical research, and Gauss curve provides a useful standardization.
- Gauss curve facilitates comparisons as well as statistical analyses.

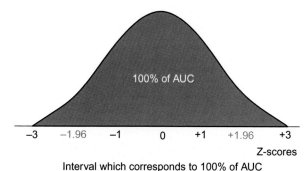

Interval which corresponds to 100% of AUC

FIGURE 8.2   The Gauss curve and its main features. AUC, area under the curve.

- It efficiently reproduces the biological characteristics of a population, which tend to present a spiked mean sided by progressively dispersed values (concentrated within standard deviation range and scarce outside of it).
- It graphically expresses the probability of finding a given value inside the studied population or sample (the closer to zero, the greater this probability).

In the following example, we illustrate how to turn the results of a trial into a Gauss curve. Arterial blood oxygen saturation (SO_2) values from a sample of 16 patients with chronic pulmonary obstructive disease (COPD), admitted to the intensive care unit (ICU) of a veterans' hospital, are detailed in Table 8.2.

The mean of this sample is 90 and standard deviation ± 1.6. The critical ratio formula yields Z-scores as detailed in Table 8.3.

By tabulating Z-scores according to the number of subjects presenting a specific arterial blood SO_2, we derive Table 8.4.

By plotting Z-scores as a Gauss curve, we derive Figure 8.3. This distribution pattern can be considered as normal.

In "real world" populations, normal distribution curves do not present themselves as evenly drawn as in the previous example. In fact, they usually show nonuniformities that may even cast doubt on their actual normality. Therefore, one can infer that the limit between normality and non-normality may not be well-defined, which may render the corresponding decision rather subjective. The following are parameters that may aid in this definition:

- Morphology of the curve (asymmetries, skewness, and kurtosis)
- Proximity in relation to mean, median, and mode (the closer among themselves, the more "normal" the curve is expected to be)

TABLE 8.2 Results of Arterial Blood SO$_2$ of a Sample of 16 Patients Admitted to the ICU

Patient No.	Arterial Blood SO$_2$ (%)
Patient 1	90
Patient 2	91
Patient 3	89
Patient 4	92
Patient 5	88
Patient 6	93
Patient 7	90
Patient 8	89
Patient 9	91
Patient 10	88
Patient 11	92
Patient 12	90
Patient 13	89
Patient 14	91
Patient 15	90
Patient 16	87

TABLE 8.3 Z-Scores of the Sample of COPD Patients from Table 8.2

Patient No.	Arterial Blood SO$_2$	Z-Score
Patient 1	90	0
Patient 2	91	0.62
Patient 3	89	− 0.62
Patient 4	92	1.25
Patient 5	88	− 1.25

(Continued)

TABLE 8.3 (Continued)

Patient No.	Arterial Blood SO$_2$	Z-Score
Patient 6	93	1.87
Patient 7	90	0
Patient 8	89	− 0.62
Patient 9	91	0.62
Patient 10	88	− 1.25
Patient 11	92	1.25
Patient 12	90	0
Patient 13	89	− 0.62
Patient 14	91	0.62
Patient 15	90	0
Patient 16	87	− 1.87

TABLE 8.4 Z-Scores Correlated to the Number of Patients with a Specific Arterial Blood SO$_2$

No. of Patients with a Specific Arterial Blood SO$_2$	Arterial Blood SO$_2$	Z-Score
4	90	0
3	91	0.62
3	89	−0.62
2	92	1.25
2	88	−1.25
1	93	1.87
1	87	−1.87

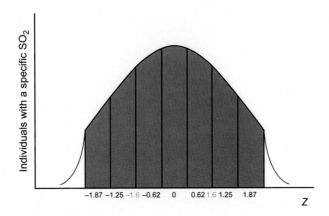

FIGURE 8.3   Graphic plotting of Z-scores corresponding to arterial blood SO_2 from the COPD patients sample.

- A 95% confidence interval (Step 7; Chapter 10) that encompasses two standard deviations
- A coefficient of variation (Step 4; Chapter 7) between 25 and 50%

Consistency or nonconsistency of study data with a normal distribution pattern will determine which might be the most suitable statistical test in order to determine p, or if $p < \alpha$. These tests are represented by two main groups: parametric (consistent with normal distribution) and nonparametric (nonconsistent with normal distribution).

APPENDIX 8.1: HOW TO VERIFY NORMALITY OF A GRAPH CURVE USING MICROSOFT EXCEL

Step 1

Tabulate your data, along with column names, and select the arrays. Click on the **Insert** tag and then on the **PivotTable** button in the **Tables** area for the **Create PivotTable** dialog box. Checkmark the **New Worksheet** circle in the **Choose where you want the PivotTable report to be placed** window field so that PivotTable is shown in another sheet. Click **OK** for a PivotTable worksheet.

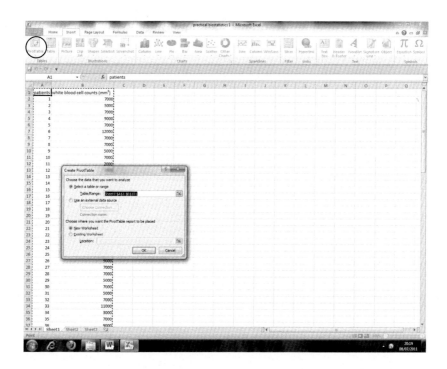

Step 2

Drag the **patients** field (do not checkmark the box) from the **Choose fields to add to report** area in the **PivotTable Field List** window to the **Σ Values** area in the **Drag fields between areas below** field (same window). Drag the **white blood cells (mm3)** field (do not checkmark the box) from the **Choose fields to add to report** area in the **PivotTable Field List** window to the **Row Labels** area in the **Drag fields between areas below** field (same window). A report is built, but notice that Excel treats patients' identification numbers as arguments by summing them up in the **Sum of Patient** column.

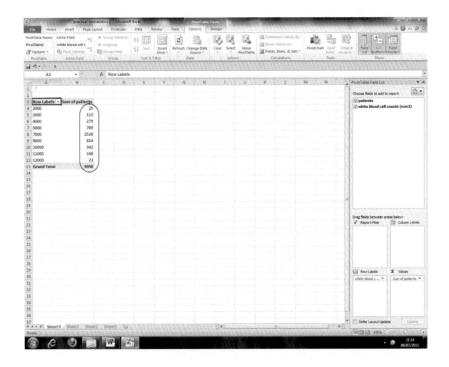

In order to correct it, click on the **Sum of Patients** field drop-down menu in the **Σ values** area and then on the **Value Field Settings** option for the **Value Field Settings** dialog box. Select the **Count Numbers** option in the **Summarize value field by** area in the **Summarize Values By** tag. Click **OK**.

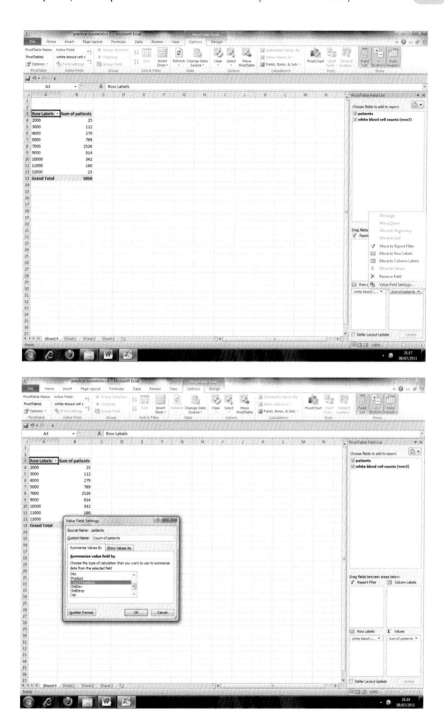

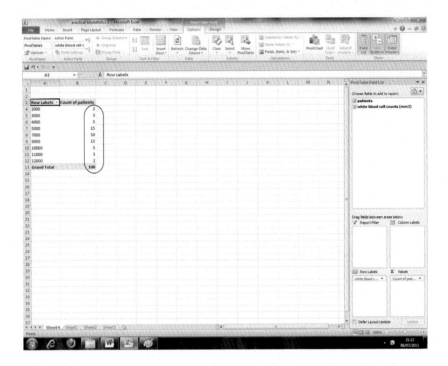

Step 3

Patients are now correctly referred to, and we can continue. Click on the **Insert** tag and then on the **Line** button in the **Charts** area for the **2-D/3-D** drop-down menu. Click on the **Line** button under the **2-D Line** option.

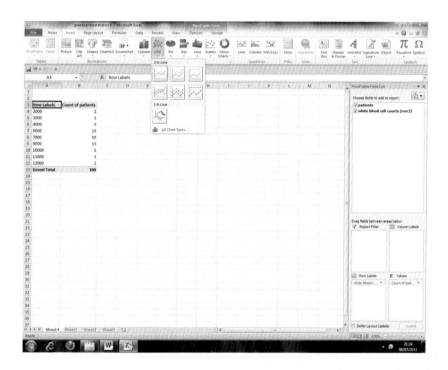

A graphical expression of your initial table is shown. If you wish, you can make your graph look as "round" as the graph shown in the third screenshot that follows. Right-click on the graph's line for a drop-down menu, and click on the **Format Data Series** option for the **Format Data Series** dialog box. Then click on the **Line Style** option, and checkmark the **Smoothed line** box. Click **Close**.

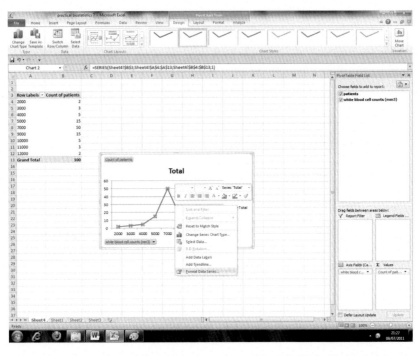

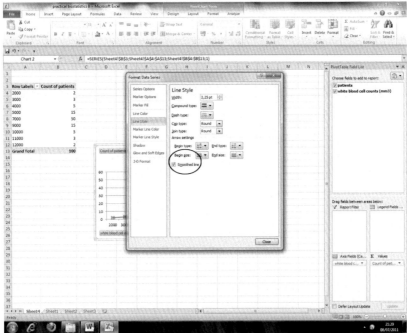

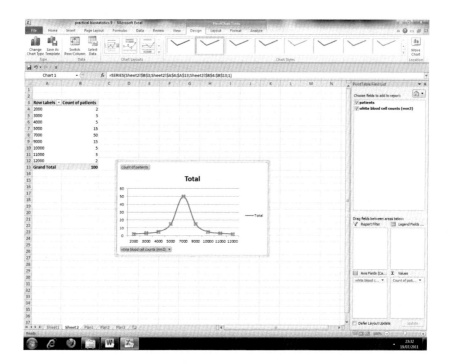

Chapter 9

Step 6: Hypothesis Testing

Hypothesis testing consists essentially of comparing central tendency and dispersal measures between two samples in order to test the investigator's hypothesis.[1] This comparison is performed using special tools called statistical tests, whose aim is to reject or not the null hypothesis (H_0, meaning the difference between measures does not achieve a statistically significant difference, according to a tabulated critical value). In this chapter, the type of measure used to demonstrate how some of these tests work is the mean.

The parameters usually followed in the process of hypothesis testing are as follows:

- Type of distribution of study data
  - Parametric tests: Parametric tests allow a safer H_0 rejection. They are called "parametric" because they are based on Gaussian parameters (mean and standard deviation) based on a normal distribution of data (Step 5; Chapter 8). The following are criteria for their applicability:
    - Samples must be independent (Chapter 1).
    - Dispersal measures between compared samples must be homogeneous.
    - Variables must be quantitative (Step 3; Chapter 6).
  - Nonparametric tests: They are called "nonparametric" because they are not based on Gaussian parameters (mean and standard deviation). Nonparametric tests are useful whenever parametric tests do not apply. They are statistically weaker, and they are applicable in the following situations:
    - There is a non-normal data distribution.
    - Different conditions prevail among individuals from the same sample.
    - Dispersal measures between compared samples are not homogeneous.
    - Qualitative variables are involved (especially ordinal variables) (Step 3; Chapter 6).
    - There is a small n.

---

[1] In fact, hypothesis testing can involve one, two, or three or more samples comparisons. In this chapter, only two-sample testing is detailed.

M. Suchmacher & M. Geller: Practical Biostatistics. DOI: 10.1016/B978-0-12-415794-1.00009-4

- Number of samples to be compared
  - One sample comparison (the sample is compared to the population from which it was taken)
  - Two samples comparison
  - Three or more samples comparison
- Degrees of freedom $(\nu)^2$
  - For calculating statistical parameters for populations or samples, one must consider the number of individual variables contained in them. These, of course, "vary"; that is, they are "free" to assume different values. Therefore, there should be as many "degrees of freedom" as individual variables. For example, if there are 10 individual variables or 10 individuals in a population, there are 10 degrees of freedom in it.
  - Due to mathematical concepts not discussed here, the number of degrees of freedom in a population coincides with its N, and for samples it corresponds to $n - 1$. In the former example, the number of degrees of freedom is 10. If these 10 individual variables belonged to a sample, then the number of degrees of freedom would be $10 - 1 = 9$.
- Statistical significance level (α) (Step 1; Chapter 4)

  An α of 0.05 is the usual statistical significance level adopted, and it is usually applied whenever one-sided hypotheses (Step 2; Chapter 3) are proposed. For example, we want to verify if A intervention (sample A) and B intervention (sample B) are capable of significantly increasing respective means, $\bar{x}_A$ and $\bar{x}_B$, in comparison with the mean of a reference sample, $\bar{x}_R$ (Figure 9.1). Most proposed hypotheses in health care sciences yield one-sided results.
- Type of relation between samples' individuals (Chapter 1)
  - Dependent samples
  - Independent samples
- Type of variables (Step 3; Chapter 6)
  - Qualitative (categorical or ordinal)
  - Quantitative (discrete or continuous)

Some parametric and nonparametric types of tests are shown in Table 9.1. Some of the most commonly applied tests are further detailed here.

For each type of test, there is a corresponding distribution table, which generally associates three parameters:

- The significance cutoff, as chosen by the investigator (α, generally 0.05)

---

[2] Pronounced as "noo."

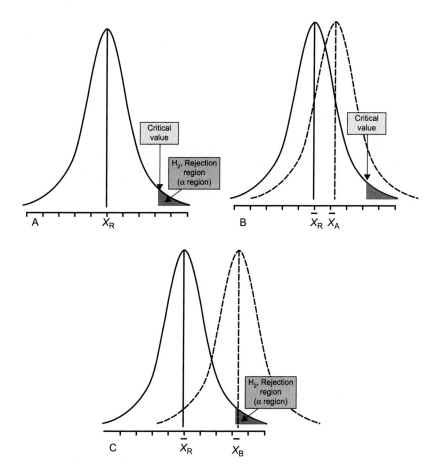

FIGURE 9.1   (A) Curve corresponding to data distribution of reference sample and $\bar{x}_R$. Critical value corresponds to the conventional statistical significance cutoff (0.05), beyond which $\bar{x}_A$ and/or $\bar{x}_B$ would enter the H_0 rejection region (α region). (B) Although $\bar{x}_A$ is greater than $\bar{x}_R$, it does not touch the critical value line. Therefore, one cannot reject H_0 (i.e., the hypothesis that there is no significant difference between reference sample and sample A means). In other words, there is no statistically significant difference between them. (C) $\bar{x}_B$ is greater than $\bar{x}_R$, and it passes the critical value line, entering the H_0 rejection region (α region). Therefore, one can reject H_0. In other words, there is a statistically significant difference between them.

- Degrees of freedom of studied samples
- Samples n

By associating these, we can find the critical value against which the statistic found by the chosen statistical test must be paired. If the test statistic is greater than the critical value, we infer that $p < \alpha$, and H_0 is rejected. If the opposite is inferred, then H_0 cannot be rejected.

TABLE 9.1 **Examples of Statistical Tests Classified According to Type of Distribution of Study Data and Type of Comparison**

Parametric		Nonparametric	
Independent	*Dependent*	*Independent*	*Dependent*
Two samples comparison			
Student's *t* test	Paired Student's *t* test	Mann–Whitney test χ^2 test	Wilcoxon signed-rank test
Two or more samples comparison			
ANOVA	ANOVA	χ^2 test	Cochran test

ANOVA = analysis of variance.

9.1 PARAMETRIC TESTS FOR INDEPENDENT AND DEPENDENT SAMPLES

9.1.1 Student's *t* Test

Student's *t* test aims to detect differences between means of samples whose data present a normal distribution. A derived statistic, *T*, is meant to be compared to a specific value in a *t* distribution table, $t_{\nu,\alpha}$, for statistical significance. *T* is calculated by the following formula:

$$T = \frac{\bar{x}_A - \bar{x}_B}{S_c^2 \sqrt{(1/n_A + 1/n_B)}}$$

where $\bar{x}_A$ is the sample A mean, $\bar{x}_B$ is the sample B mean, S_c^2 is the combined variance from samples A and B (formula not detailed here), n_A is the sample A *n*, and n_B is the sample B *n*.

Degrees of freedom is calculated as follows:

$$\nu = (n_A + n_B) - 2$$

For example, 30 patients with hypertriglyceridemia were randomized between two different therapeutic regimens: sample A, comprising 15 patients with lipid-lowering diet only, and sample B, comprising 15 patients with lipid-lowering diet plus oral gemfibrozil. The following is the investigator's hypothesis: Could oral gemfibrozil increase triglyceride-lowering properties of a lipid-lowering diet?

H_0: Diet plus oral gemfibrozil does not lower triglyceride serum levels better than diet only.
H_1: Diet plus oral gemfibrozil lowers serum triglyceride levels better than diet only.

TABLE 9.2 *n* and Statistics of Samples A and B

	Sample A	Sample B
n	15	15
Triglyceride $\bar{x}$	150	135
Standard deviation	33.6	32.4

TABLE 9.3 Reproduction of Part of a *t* Distribution Table

Degrees of Freedom (*v*)		α	
	0.025	*0.05*	*0.10*
25	2.060	1.708	1.316
26	2.056	1.706	1.315
27	2.052	1.703	1.314
28	2.048	**1.701**	1.313
29	2.045	1.699	1.311

Mean and standard deviations of both samples are tabulated (Table 9.2). *T* and degrees of freedom are calculated as follows:

$$T = \frac{150 - 135}{33.06\sqrt{(0.13)}} = 1.27$$
$$v = (15 + 15) - 2 = 28$$

A *t* distribution table is consulted for the critical value corresponding to $t_{28,0.05}$ (part of this table is shown in Table 9.3).

We learn that $T = 1.27 < t_{28,0.05} = 1.701$; that is, although there is a difference between serum triglyceride levels between these samples, it is not significant from a statistical perspective. In other words, we are not authorized to reject H_0.

9.1.2 Paired Student's *t* Test

Paired Student's *t* test aims to detect differences between means of the same sample, before and after an intervention (a "self-paired" sample). A derived statistic *T* is meant to be compared to a specific value in a *t* distribution table, $t_{\nu,\alpha}$, for statistical significance. T is determined by the following formula:

$$T = \frac{\bar{d}}{S_{\mathbf{d}}/\sqrt{n}}$$

where $\bar{d}$ is the before and after difference between means, and $S_{\mathbf{d}}$ is the standard deviation of the difference (**d**) between individual values.

Degrees of freedom is calculated as follows:

$$\nu = n - 1$$

For example, the same sample of 10 emergency room (ER) patients with acute respiratory failure under artificial ventilation was tested before and after the use of an aerosolized bronchodilator. The following is the investigator's hypothesis: Could an aerosolized bronchodilator increase tidal volume in the same sample of ER patients with acute respiratory failure under artificial ventilation?

H_0: Artificial ventilation plus aerosolized bronchodilator does not increase tidal volume better than artificial ventilation only in the same sample of ER patients with acute respiratory failure.

H_1: Artificial ventilation plus aerosolized bronchodilator increases tidal volume better than artificial ventilation only in a sample of ER patients with acute respiratory failure.

Results are detailed in Table 9.4.

TABLE 9.4 Results of Tidal Volumes Before and After Tested Treatment

Patient No.	Before	After	d^a
1	620	620	0
2	710	720	−10
3	850	870	−20
4	750	765	−15
5	600	625	−25
6	550	590	−40
7	620	620	0
8	690	750	−60
9	790	810	−20
10	790	805	−15

[a]Difference.

$$\bar{x}_{\text{before}} = 697$$
$$\bar{x}_{\text{after}} = 718$$
$$\bar{d} = 718 - 697 = 21$$
$$S_d = 18.1$$
$$T = \frac{21}{18.1/\sqrt{10}} = 3.75$$
$$\nu = 10 - 1 = 9$$

A t distribution table is consulted for the critical value corresponding to $t_{9,0.05}$. We learn that $T = 3.75 > t_{9,0.05} = 2.262$ (the critical value); that is, the difference between tidal volumes before and after aerosolized bronchodilator is statistically significant. In other words, we are authorized to reject H_0 with a 5% probability of being wrong ($p_\alpha < 0.05$).

9.2 NONPARAMETRIC TESTS

Nonparametric tests often involve value ranking rather than the measured value itself.

9.2.1 For Independent Samples

Mann–Whitney Test

The Mann–Whitney test aims to detect differences of variable values between two samples through ranking. A derived statistic, U or U', is meant to be compared to a specific value in a Mann–Whitney distribution table, $U_{\alpha,n1,n2}$ or $U_{\alpha,n2,n1}$, for statistical significance. If $n1 > n2$, then U or U' is compared against $U_{\alpha,n1,n2}$; if $n2 > n1$, then it is compared against $U_{\alpha,n2,n1}$ (note that comparisons performed in such a way are applicable only to two-sided tests). U and U' are determined by the following formulas, respectively:

$$U = n_1 \times n_2 + \frac{n_1 \times (n_1 + 1)}{2} - R_1$$
$$U' = n_1 \times n_2 - U$$

where n_1 is the number of individuals in sample 1, n_2 is the number of individuals in sample 2, and R_1 is the sum of sample 1 ranks.

For example, 12 patients with chronic pain were randomized between two different analgesic regimens: sample 1, paracetamol, and sample 2, paracetamol plus codeine. The following is the investigator's hypothesis: Could codeine significantly increase the analgesic properties of paracetamol?

H_0: Codeine does not increase the analgesic properties of paracetamol.
H_1: Codeine increases the analgesic properties of paracetamol.

Results are detailed in Tables 9.5 and 9.6.

TABLE 9.5 Ranked Results for Pain Levels for Sample 1

Sample 1 Patients ($n1$)	Pain Level (VAS)[a]	Rank[b]
1	43	11th
2	40	12th
3	50	9th
4	45	10th
5	59	7th
6	56	8th
7	79	4th
		$R_1 = 61$

[a]Visual analogic scale (0–100 mm).
[b]Ranked from the smallest to the largest variable value.

TABLE 9.6 Ranked Results for Pain Levels for Sample 2

Sample 2 Patients ($n2$)	Pain Level (VAS)[a]	Rank[b]
1	77	5th
2	60	6th
3	90	2nd
4	81	3rd
5	92	1st
		$R_2 = 17$

[a]Visual analogic scale (0–100 mm).
[b]Ranked from the smallest to the largest variable value.

$$U = 7 \times 5 + \frac{7 \times (7 + 1)}{2} - 61 = 2$$

$$U' = 7 \times 5 - 2 = 33$$

$$U_{\alpha,n1,n2} = U_{0.05,7,5} = 30 \ \text{(critical value)}$$

A Mann–Whitney distribution table is consulted for the critical value corresponding to $U_{0.05,7,5}$. We learn that $U' = 33 > U_{0.05,7,5} = 30$ (the critical value); that is, the difference between pain levels of these samples is statistically significant. In other words, we are authorized to reject H_0 with a 5% probability of being wrong ($p_\alpha < 0.05$).

χ^2 Test

The χ^2 test aims to find event rate differences between two or more samples, studied as categorical variables plotted in a two-by-two contingency table (only its applicability between two samples is depicted here). χ^2 is determined by the following formula:

$$\chi^2 = \frac{\sum (\text{observed rate} - \text{expected rate})^2}{\text{expected rate}}$$

Degrees of freedom is determined as follows:

$$\nu = (\text{lines number} - 1) \times (\text{columns number} - 1)$$

For example, 209 patients in acute lymphoid leukemia (ALL) first remission were randomized between two different chemotherapy protocols: protocol 1 and protocol 2. After 1 year, remission and relapse rates are determined. The following is the investigator's hypothesis: Would there be significant differences between protocol 1 and protocol 2 remission and relapse rates?

H_0: There are no significant differences between protocol 1 and protocol 2 remission and relapse rates.

H_1: There are significant differences between protocol 1 and protocol 2 remission and relapse rates.

Results are detailed in Table 9.7.

To address this hypothesis, we must first estimate the expected remission and relapse rates − as if there is no therapeutic influence − using a simple rule of three:

● Subgroup A: From a total of 209 patients, 102 remained in remission. From a subtotal of 72 patients treated with protocol 1, 35.1 remissions would therefore be expected.
● Subgroup B: From a total of 209 patients, 107 relapsed. From a subtotal of 72 patients treated with protocol 1, 36.8 relapses would therefore be expected.
● Subgroup C: From a total of 209 patients, 102 remained in remission. From a subtotal of 137 patients treated with protocol 2, 66.8 remissions would therefore be expected.

TABLE 9.7 ALL Patients in Remission and Relapse, According to Protocol

	In Remission	In Relapse	Total
Protocol 1 patients	21 (subgroup A)	51 (subgroup B)	72
Protocol 2 patients	81 (subgroup C)	56 (subgroup D)	137
Total	102	107	209

- Subgroup D: From a total of 209 patients, 107 relapsed. From a subtotal of 137 patients treated with protocol 2, 70.1 relapses would therefore be expected.

$$\chi^2 = \frac{(21 - 35.1)^2}{35.1} + \frac{(51 - 36.8)^2}{36.8} + \frac{(81 - 66.8)^2}{66.8} + \frac{(56 - 70.1)^2}{70.1} = 17$$

$$\nu = (2 - 1) \times (2 - 1) = 1$$

A χ^2 distribution table is consulted for the critical value (assuming $\alpha = 0.05$ and $\nu = 1$). We learn that $\chi^2 = 17 > 3.841$ (the critical value); that is, the difference between protocol 1 and protocol 2 remission and relapse rates after 1 year is statistically significant. In other words, we are authorized to reject H_0 with a 5% probability of being wrong ($p_\alpha < 0.05$). Because most protocol 2 patients remained in remission after 1 year, and most protocol 1 patients did not, we can infer that protocol 2 yields better therapeutic results compared to protocol 1 (note that the χ^2 test is applicable only if observed rates are >20 and expected rates are >5).

9.2.2 For Dependent Samples: Wilcoxon Signed-Rank Test

The Wilcoxon signed-rank test aims to detect differences between variables from the same sample before and after an intervention by calculating the differences between their ranks. A derived statistic, T, is compared to a specific value in a T distribution table, $T_{\alpha,n}$, for statistical significance. Pre- and post-intervention differences are calculated, ranked, and summed as $T+$ and $T-$.

For example, the same sample of 10 patients with paroxysmal coughing was tested before and after the administration of an experimental cough medicine. The following is the investigator's hypothesis: Could this experimental cough medicine improve paroxysmal coughing according to a cough-related quality-of-life questionnaire (CQLQ) in the same sample of patients?

H_0: Experimental cough medicine does not improve paroxysmal coughing.
H_1: Experimental cough medicine improves paroxysmal coughing.

Results are detailed in Table 9.8.

$T+$ (all $+$ signed-ranks are summed) $= 51$
$T-$ (all $-$ signed-ranks are summed) $= 4$

A T distribution table is consulted for the critical value corresponding to $T_{\alpha,n}$. We learn that $T_{0.05,10} = 8$ (the critical value) $> T- = 4$; that is, the difference between pre- and post-treatment CQLQ scores with the experimental cough medicine is statistically significant (note that $T+$ could have also been used if it were smaller than $T_{\alpha,n}$). In other words, we are authorized to reject H_0 with a 5% probability of being wrong ($p_\alpha < 0.05$).

TABLE 9.8 Ranked Changes in Pre- and Post-Treatment with the Experimental Cough Medicine, with Corresponding Differences

Patient No.	Pretreatment Score[a]	Post-Treatment Score[a]	Difference[b]	Difference Rank[c]	DIfference Signed-Rank[d]
1	140	136	4 (4th)	4.5	4.5
2	142	138	4 (5th)	4.5	4.5
3	144	139	5 (8th)	7	7
4	144	147	−3 (3rd)	3	−3
5	146	141	5 (6th)	7	7
6	142	143	−1 (1st)	1	−1
7	150	145	5 (7th)	7	7
8	149	143	6 (9th)	9.5	9.5
9	148	146	2 (2nd)	2	2
10	142	136	6 (10th)	9.5	9.5

[a]Sum of CQLQ parameters.
[b]Ranked from smallest to largest difference.
[c]Calculated according to rank difference, not to the difference itself; where ranks coincide with equal differences, the corresponding means are represented by decimal values.
[d]Difference signal is assigned to rank.

Chapter 10

Step 7: Correlating Sample Data with the General Population – 95% Confidence Interval

After determining if there is a statistically significant difference between study group and control group endpoint values, it is necessary to extrapolate corresponding results to the general population because it would not be useful for health sciences to collect data that would be applicable only to the studied sample. This correlation is established through the determination of *sample statistics*, generally expressed as a percentage corresponding to a conventional interval – *confidence interval* – found in a normal distribution graph.

One of the principles that allows estimations from a sample to population is that *a sample preserves the same random distribution of variable values as that of the population from which it was taken*. For example, suppose we have a 1000 L water tank containing a population of 3000 fish that swim at random speeds and in random directions (our variables). Then, we sample 10 L from this tank. The sample contains 30 fish in a fish bowl, which also swim at random speeds and in random directions. Although it is just a sample, it does preserve the same randomness of the original population. Assuming that we do not have access to the data for the whole tank, we need to learn how to "amplify" the randomness of the fish bowl, expressed by its variables, in order to infer the "big picture."

This "amplification" is feasible, and it is based on three fundamental concepts: *sampling distribution*, *central limit theorem*, and *probability theory*. Sampling distribution consists of distributing a population into samples (with each sample containing the same number of individuals), as in the example depicted in Figure 10.1.

Sampling distribution is the basis of two estimation methods: *point estimation* and *interval estimation*.

M. Suchmacher & M. Geller: Practical Biostatistics. DOI: 10.1016/B978-0-12-415794-1.00010-0

10.1 POINT ESTIMATION

Point estimation consists of estimating *population mean* (μ) and *population standard deviation* (σ) based on the so-called *estimators* — that is, *sample mean* ($\bar{x}$) and *standard error of the mean* ($S_{\bar{x}}$), respectively. Some of the statistical principles that support this proposal are detailed here.

10.1.1 Sampling Distribution of the Mean and the Sampling Mean

Sampling distribution of the mean (actually sampling distribution of the means because it refers to two or more means) consists of distributing the means of each sample of the *sampling distribution* (it is understood that each sample is composed of a fixed *n*) (Figure 10.2).

According to the central limit theorem,[1] if we plotted these sample means on a graph, the resulting curve would tend to appear as a normal distribution. The shape of this curve would basically depend on the following two factors:

- Number of sample means: The more sample means we plot, the more "normal" this curve would appear.

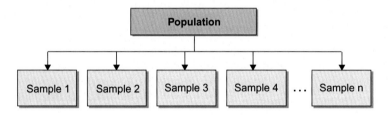

FIGURE 10.1   *Sampling distribution* of a population.

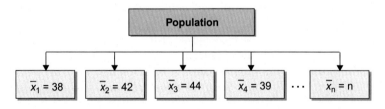

FIGURE 10.2   *Sampling distribution of the mean* in Figure 10.1, with exemplifying figures.

---

[1] The central limit theorem establishes the principles on which sample means of a sufficiently large number of samples containing a uniform number of variables, extracted from the same population, yield a normal or close to normal distribution despite the randomness of this sampling.

- Number of individuals per each sample: The more individuals per sample, the narrower this curve would appear.

Sampling mean ($\mu_{\bar{x}}$) corresponds to the mean of all the means of the sampling distribution of the mean, according to the following formula:

$$\mu_{\bar{x}} = \frac{\bar{x}_1 + \bar{x}_2 + \bar{x}_3 + \bar{x}_4 + \ldots + \bar{x}_n}{\text{number of samples}}$$

According to probability theory, sampling mean tends to be equal to population mean. We can intuitively assume that the greater the n of the samples of this sampling mean, the closer sampling mean is to *population mean*. This assumption allows us to estimate population mean based on the mean of a given sample.

Based on the previous assumptions, and on probability theory (detailed elsewhere), it is possible to propose the number of individuals per sample for population mean estimation, using the sample mean as an estimator:

- The population presents a normal distribution.
  Plotting all sample means would result in a normal distribution curve, regardless of the number of individuals per sample.
- The population does not present a normal distribution.
  Plotting all sample means would result in a normal distribution curve if there are 30 or more individuals per sample. If the distribution pattern of the population is not known (as is often the case), it is advisable to assume it is not normal in order to increase the probability that, in our study, *sample mean = population mean*.

Intuitively, it is reasonable to propose that if the population presents a normal distribution of data, the least the number of individuals per sample and the number of sample means necessary in order to build up a normal distribution curve based on the sample means. Conversely, if the population does not present a normal distribution, the greater the number of individuals per sample and the number of sample means necessary in order to obtain the same result.

10.1.2 Standard Error

Standard error ($\sigma_{\bar{x}}$) is an estimation of the standard deviation of the sampling distribution of the mean. It is calculated by the following formula:

$$\sigma_{\bar{x}} = \frac{\sigma}{\sqrt{n}}$$

where σ is the population standard deviation, and n is the number of individuals in the sample.

Two points are inferable from this equation:

- The wider the population standard deviation, the wider the standard error. This means that the standard error tends to follow the population standard deviation.
- The greater the number of individuals per sample, the narrower the standard error. This means that (1) the difference between standard error and population standard deviation tends to be smaller, and (2) the difference between sample mean and population mean tends to be smaller.

The limitation of standard error is that, in practice, we seldom know the population standard deviation.

10.1.3 Standard Error of the Mean

Standard error of the mean ($S_{\bar{x}}$) (Step 4; Chapter 7) is an alternative way to estimate the standard deviation of the sampling distribution of the mean, using sample standard deviation instead of population standard deviation. It is calculated by the following formula:

$$S_{\bar{x}} = \frac{S}{\sqrt{n}}$$

where S is the sample standard deviation, and n is the number of individuals in the sample.

Two points are inferable from this equation:

- The wider the sample standard deviation, the wider the standard error of the mean. This means that the standard error of the mean tends to follow the sample standard deviation.
- The greater the number of individuals per sample, the narrower the standard error of the mean. This means that there is a smaller the difference between the standard error of the mean and the standard deviation of the sampling distribution of the mean.

In the standard error of the mean equation, the variable sample standard deviation has to be determined or estimated by the statistician. However, because we are dealing with samples and not with populations (as in standard error), this would be a less problematic task. Based on the previous assumptions, and on probability theory, it is possible to propose the standard error of the mean as an estimator for population standard deviation.

Hence, by determining sample mean and standard error of the mean, it is possible to estimate population mean and population standard deviation, respectively, on a probability basis (complete methodology detailed elsewhere).

10.2 INTERVAL ESTIMATION (95% CONFIDENCE INTERVAL)

Although point estimation provides a solid probability basis for sample-to-population extrapolations, a precise coincidence between a sample estimator and corresponding population parameter would be an unlikely event, at least in clinical research. The idea of interval estimation is to widen the probability that the statistic found in the studied sample might coincide with the parameter of the general population by building a conventional interval siding this statistic. Let us adopt the graph from Step 5 (Chapter 8, Figure 8.2) as an example, and assume that it derives from a hypothetical original sample (Figure 10.3).

Based on the graph, the following points can be inferred:

- The closer to the mean a given sample value is, the greater the probability for its detection in the general population.
- α represents the statistical significance level that corresponds to the highest tolerable cutoff for a type I error (Step 1; Chapter 4). If we assume an α of 5% regarding the statement that all the values in a sample can be found in the general population (i.e., a 5% probability that this statement is not true), for inference there would remain a 95% confidence that such a statement is true. In other words, there would be a 95% probability of finding a given sample value in the general population and a 5% probability of not finding it. This assumption can be expressed by the following formula:

$$100\% - \alpha = 95\%$$

Hence, 95% would correspond to a conventional confidence level. Assuming that the farther a sample value is from sample mean, the lesser the probability of finding it in the general population, then the values corresponding to α are supposed to be found in the upper and lower extremities

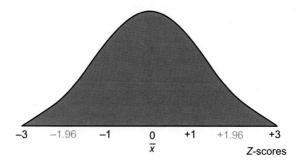

FIGURE 10.3   Example of a normal distribution curve, with Z-scores ($\bar{x}$ = mean).

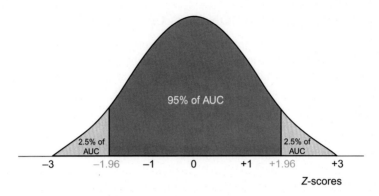

FIGURE 10.4 The area under the curve (AUC) and interval corresponding to the probability of finding a sample statistic (or endpoint value) in the general population. If we assume that the probability of 95% in finding a sample value in the general population is two-tailed and symmetrical, then we must also distribute α symmetrically; that is, $\alpha/2 = 2.5\%$ per tail.

of the sample's value range. By expressing the latter inference graphically, we would derive Figure 10.4.

By convention, we place our "confidence" in the theory that the statistic found under the sample's 95% area under the curve (AUC) might coincide with the corresponding parameter eventually found in the general population. According to Gauss curve, 95% of AUC corresponds to the interval between Z-scores, -1.96 to $+1.96$ standard deviation (SD). Hence, this interval is called the 95% confidence interval (95% CI).

The SDs of -1.96 and $+1.96$ correspond to inferior and superior confidence limits of a sample, respectively. In order to determine them, we can apply the confidence limits formula:

$$x_i = \bar{x} - 1.96 \cdot S_{\bar{x}}$$
$$x_s = \bar{x} + 1.96 \cdot S_{\bar{x}}$$

where x_s is the superior confidence limit, x_i is the inferior confidence limit, $\bar{x}$ = mean, and $S_{\bar{x}}$ (standard error of the mean) = $S/\sqrt{n}$ (where S is the sample standard deviation, and n is the number of individuals in the sample) (Step 4; Chapter 7).

Actually, these formulas are better applicable for a sample related to a population whose population standard deviation is unknown. However, if the latter is unknown (as in fact it is in most cases), it is licit to replace population standard deviation for sample standard deviation in the numerator of the standard error of the mean part of the equation if n is large enough (roughly ≥ 30 individuals). This is due to the fact that sample standard deviation tends to approximate population standard deviation as n enlarges.

Let us check two examples taken from two different samples of mild renal failure patients containing 32 individuals each:

- Sample A

  $\bar{x}$ is equal to 80 mL/min of creatinine clearance, and S is equal to ± 51. Applying the confidence limits formula, we have:

$$x_i = 80 - 1.96 \left(\frac{51}{\sqrt{32}} \right) = 62.0 \text{ mL/min}$$

$$x_s = 80 + 1.96 \left(\frac{51}{\sqrt{32}} \right) = 98.0 \text{ mL/min}$$

Hence, we can state that sample A has a 95% CI of 62.0–98 mL/min. This means that one has a 95% confidence that a randomly selected individual from a population of patients with a clinical picture of mild renal failure might present a creatinine clearance value inside this range (the closer to $\bar{x}$ − 80 mL/min − the greater the probability).

- Sample B

  $\bar{x}$ is equal to 80 mL/min of creatinine clearance, and S is equal to ± 34. Applying the confidence limits formula, we have:

$$x_i = 80 - 1.96 \left(\frac{34}{\sqrt{32}} \right) = 68.0 \text{ mL/min}$$

$$x_s = 80 + 1.96 \left(\frac{34}{\sqrt{32}} \right) = 92.0 \text{ mL/min}$$

Hence, we can state that sample B has a 95% CI of 68.0–92.0 mL/min. This means that one has a 95% confidence that a randomly selected individual from a population of patients with a clinical picture of mild renal failure might present a creatinine clearance value inside this range (the closer to $\bar{x}$ − 80 mL/min − the greater the probability).

By graphically plotting the data from sample A and sample B, we obtain Figure 10.5.

Thus, if we have two 95% CIs, which one can we put our "confidence" in the most? The answer depends on the objective of the study. Let us analyze two possible interpretations inferable from each sample:

- Sample A

  Because it has a more heterogeneous population from a biological standpoint, it generates a wider standard deviation and consequently a wider 95% CI. This sample represents the biological reality of creatinine

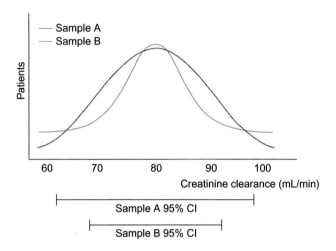

FIGURE 10.5   Superimposed 95% confidence intervals (CIs) for sample A and sample B.

clearance in the context of mild renal failure more poorly because its population is so heterogeneous. On the other hand, corresponding 95% CI can be generalized to the general population of patients with mild renal failure more promptly because such a heterogeneity is expected to be found in a "real world" context.

- Sample B
  Because it has a more homogeneous population from a biological standpoint, it generates a narrower standard deviation and consequently a narrower 95% CI. This sample better represents the biological reality of creatinine clearance in the context of mild renal failure because its population is so homogeneous. On the other hand, corresponding 95% CI cannot be generalized to the general population of patients with mild renal failure so promptly because such a homogeneity is not expected to be found in a "real world" context.

Summarizing the Steps

All contents described in Part 3 can be summarized as follows:
  The investigator. . .
- Step 1: Formulates a hypothesis
- Step 2: Selects the most adequate study type for addressing his or her hypothesis
- Step 3: Estimates n
- Step 4: Determines and organizes the variables and endpoints of the study
- Step 5: Determines collected data normality or non-normality
- Step 6: Calculates the summarizing mathematical parameters relative to study data
- Step 7: Selects the best statistical test type in order to either refute or confirm the investigator's hypothesis
- Step 8: Correlates the data of the sample with the general population; 95% CI is determined

  The above sequence is not suitable to address all types of investigator's hypotheses. For different types of investigation lines, we propose other resources, detailed in Part 4.

APPENDIX 10.1: HOW TO DETERMINE CONFIDENCE INTERVALS USING MICROSOFT EXCEL (SAMPLE A)

Step 1

Select a random cell (in this example, A1). Click on the **Formulas** tag and then on the **More Functions** button in the **Function Library** area. Click on the **Statistical** drop-down menu button and then on the **CONFIDENCE. NORM** (NORMal distribution) secondary drop-down menu button for the **Function Arguments** dialog box. The confidence interval formula is shown in the A1 cell.

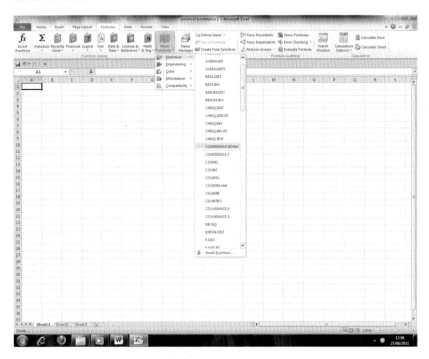

Step 2

The following arguments must be inserted in the **Function Arguments** dialog box fields: (1) alpha, 0.05; (2) standard deviation, 51; and (3) size, 32. The confidence limit is shown in the result space (you must sum and subtract it from the mean in order to obtain 95% CI).

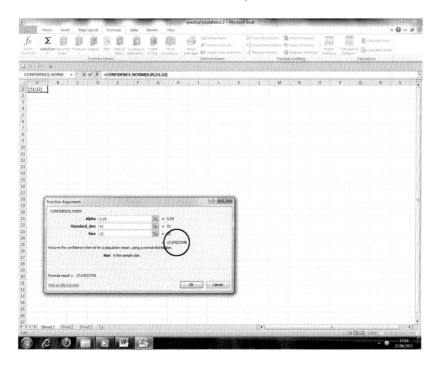

Part III Reader Resources

SELF-EVALUATION

1. "A cohort of 110 overweight patients with low back pain was assessed through a randomized study with the aim of determining efficacy and safety of a pain-killer drug. Symptom was measured with the aid of a visual analogic scale (VAS), graded from 0 (no pain) to 10 (worst pain possible)."
The type of variable corresponding to VAS was:
   A. Continuous, quantitative
   B. Discrete, quantitative
   C. Nondicotomic, categorical
   D. Ordinal, qualitative
2. Find the correct correspondence:
   1. χ^2 test
   2. Independent sample
   3. Paired Student's t test
   4. Student's t test
   5. Wilcoxon signed-rank test

   a. Individuals from a sample do not relate to individuals from a different sample.
   b. Nonparametric test for comparison of two samples with the use of a two-by-two contingency table.
   c. Parametric test for comparison of two dependent samples, which aims to find differences before and after an intervention.
   d. Parametric test for arithmetic mean comparison between two independent samples.
   e. Ranked variables are used to compare the same individuals in "before versus after" settings.
   A. 1−a, 2−d, 3−e, 4−c, 5−b
   B. 1−b, 2−a, 3−c, 4−d, 5−e
   C. 1−b, 2−a, 3−c, 4−e, 5−d
   D. 1−e, 2−a, 3−c, 4−d, 5−b
3. Read the following study abstract and then answer the question.

   We investigated the effects of online intermittent hemodiafiltration (IHDF) on lactate venous serum levels in the setting of chronic renal failure with increased anion gap metabolic acidosis, comparatively to intermittent hemodialysis (IH) (considered as gold standard procedure) in 44 patients (22 treated with IHDF and 22 with IH). Before treatment, mean venous serum lactate levels for both groups were 92 mg/dL (SD ± 35). Clinically significant effect size was established as 25 mg/dL. After a three-session schedule, lactate venous serum *levels were the following: (a) IHDF group, 76 mg/dL (SD ±1); (b) IH group, 65 mg/dL (SD ±11). We concluded that IHDF was as effective as IH in correcting lactate venous serum levels, in the setting of chronic renal failure with increased anion gap metabolic acidosis (p<0.05).*

What would be the estimate power of the statistical test applied in this study?
A. 0.60
B. 0.70
C. 0.80
D. 0.90

4. Re-read the abstract from Question 3. If the biostatistician determined a test power of 0.90 for finding a difference between IHDF and IH groups, what approximate *n* would be necessary for each?
A. 33
B. 43
C. 50
D. 52

5. Mark the correct affirmative regarding parametric or nonparametric test choice:
A. Dispersal measures between compared samples do not have to be homogeneous for parametric test application.
B. Nonparametric and parametric tests are suitable for determining *p*, regardless of *n* of trial.
C. Nonparametric tests allow for a safer null hypothesis rejection.
D. Parametric tests are based on mean and standard deviation parameters.

6. Observe the following graph and then answer the question:

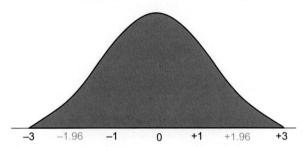

Mark the incorrect affirmative:
A. It is feasible to directly apply the original results of a given study to a distribution graph.
B. The previous graph represents a normal distribution curve, and it suggests that the most suitable statistical tests for analyzing its corresponding data are parametric tests.

    C. The morphology of this curve corresponds to Gauss curve, which approximately reproduces the characteristics of a biological population (a spiked mean sided by progressively dispersed values).

    D. Z-score interval from -1.96 SD to $+1.96$ SD corresponds to 95% of the area under the curve.

7. Read the following study abstract and then answer the question.

We studied three groups of patients with indwelling urinary catheter under long-term oral prophylactic antibiotics, with the aim of comparing colony-forming unit (CFU) concentration through urinary cultures after a 3-month period: group A (n = 40, control), group B (n = 55, norfloxacin 400 mg daily), and group C (n = 62, sulfamethoxazol–trimethoprim). Results: group A, 1,000,000 ± 20,000 CFU/mL; group B, 10,000 ± 1200 CFU/mL; and group C, 10,000 ± 500 CFU/mL. We concluded that long-term oral prophylactic antibiotics significantly decreased the concentration of CFU after a 3-month period (p < 0.05).

Mark the incorrect affirmative:

    A. Standard deviation and *n* influence the standard error of the mean (SEM) of a group, relative to the total population of a study.

    B. Because norfloxacin and sulfamethoxazol–trimethoprim yielded similar results concerning CFU urinary concentration, both probably had the same clinical efficacy.

    C. The SEM of group B is 162 and the SEM of group C is 63; therefore, group C probably represents a more homogeneous population than group B, from a biological standpoint.

    D. Coefficient of variation of group B is 12%; therefore, it represents a low dispersal coefficient of variation.

8. Mark the incorrect affirmative regarding probability in biostatistics:

    A. A type II error corresponds to the inference that a given correlation found in a scientific study is casual when in fact it is not.

    B. The null hypothesis (H_0) implies that any observed correlation is, in principle, a casual occurrence.

    C. To conclude that a given test drug is effective, with $p<0.05$, means that there is a 5% probability that the drug is actually not effective.

    D. α corresponds to the statistical significance level related to the highest tolerable cutoff for type II error.

9. Read the following study summary and then answer the question.

Two groups of unprotected patients (group A, n = 120; group B, n = 112) continuously exposed to high sound levels in their labor environment (group A, cargo area airport workers; group B, metallurgic industry workers) during a 5-year period were compared with the aim of determining high pitch frequency range (6000–7000 Hz) hearing compromise with the aid of audiogram tests.

Statistical data ($\bar{x}$, arithmetic mean; S, standard deviation) are as follows: group A, $\bar{x} = 60$ dB, S = 12; and group B, $\bar{x} = 58$ dB, S = 9.

Mark the incorrect affirmative:

A. A narrower confidence interval suggests a more homogeneous sample from a biological standpoint.

B. The 95% confidence interval (95% CI) of audiogram test results of group A ranges from 56 to 64 dB.

C. It is expected that the audiogram test results of group B (95% CI, 56.5−59.5 dB) are to be found in the general population of metallurgic industry workers exposed to similar conditions, with a 95% degree of confidence.

D. There is a 5% probability of finding audiogram test results under the inferior confidence limit of 95% CI in the general population of exposed metallurgic industry workers.

10. Mark the incorrect affirmative:

A. A sample preserves the same random distribution of variable values as the population from which it was taken.

B. One of the main objectives of hypothesis tests is to verify whether the mean of a test sample does or does not reach the H_0 (null hypothesis) rejection region of reference sample.

C. Point estimation and confidence interval are tools used for hypothesis testing between two samples.

D. Statistical significance level and number of samples to be compared are two parameters used in the process of hypothesis testing.

ANNOTATED ANSWERS

1. D. Continuous quantitative variables correspond to values expressed as whole numbers with equal intervals, possibly including fractions (e.g. 50.2 kg). Discrete quantitative variables correspond to values expressed as whole numbers with equal intervals, which do not admit fractions (e.g. 32 episodes of generalized epilepsy). Nondicotomic categorical variables correspond to qualitative values that do not admit ordering and present more than one category (e.g. sharp, burning, or throbbing pain). Ordinal qualitative variables correspond to qualitative values that admit ordering but with nonquantifiable interval sizes. Because VAS is a subjective type of graduation, determining intervals between two immediately consecutive values in a precise form is not possible.

2. B.

3. B. In order to estimate test power, and hence to assess whether the applied *n* was suitable to answer the investigator's hypothesis, it is

possible to consult a sample size nomogram. First, however, we must know the standardized difference for the adopted endpoint, which can be derived using the following formula:

$$\text{Standardized difference} = \frac{\text{target difference}}{\text{standard deviation}}$$

Target difference—the minimal effect size considered as clinically relevant by the investigators of this study—was 25 mg/dL for lactate venous serum levels, and standard deviation in the context of this sample was ±35 mg/dL. Therefore, standardized difference is approximately 0.7. By applying a sample size nomogram built for $p < 0.05$ (type I error probability chosen for this study):

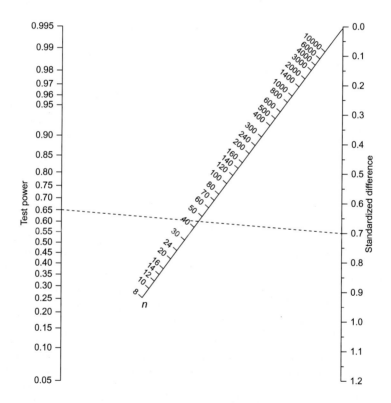

Estimate test power is therefore 0.65. By convention, the power of a biostatistical test in finding differences between two compared groups must be 80% (or 0.80). Hence, n of 44 would not, in principle, afford enough power for the test to find a difference between IHDF and IH groups.

4. B. For estimating $n_i - n$ of an individual group, we can apply the following formula:

$$n_i = \frac{2}{d^2} \cdot C_{p,power}$$

where n_i is the n of an individual group, d is the standardized difference, and $C_{p,power}$ is the constant defined by p and test power. $C_{p,power}$ can be determined according to the following table:

P	Test Power			
	50	80	90	95
0.05	3.8	7.9	10.5	13.0

$$n_i = \frac{2}{0.7^2} \cdot 10.5 = 43$$

5. D. Parametric tests demand that dispersal measures of compared samples be homogeneous. Rejecting H_0 for smaller n trials is better accomplished with nonparametric tests. Actually, parametric tests, rather than nonparametric tests, are the ones that allow for a safer H_0 rejection. Parametric tests are called "parametric" because they are based on the parameters of mean and standard deviation.

6. A. Before applying the original results of a study to a distribution graph, it is necessary to convert them to Z-scores using the critical ratio formula:

$$Z = \frac{x - \bar{x}}{S}$$

where x is the collected study value, $\bar{x}$ is the mean, and S is the standard deviation of the sample.

7. B. Because groups B and C have different n and standard deviations, and therefore different standard errors of the mean, it would be difficult to infer comparative efficacy data in the setting of this study. In order to obtain more reliable results concerning this outcome, a second study would probably be necessary.

8. D. The finding that p is equal to or lower than α authorizes the investigator to reject H_0 (the null hypothesis) and to accept H_1 (the alternative hypothesis). By doing so, the probability for type I error (not type II) — that is, that the found correlation is actually casual — diminishes to a conventional value inferior to 5%.

9. D. By convention, there would be a 2.5% — not 5% — probability of finding audiogram test results under the inferior confidence limit of 95% CI, from group A or group B, in the general population of metallurgic industry workers. By inference, there would be a 2.5% probability

of finding audiogram test results over the superior confidence limit of 95% CI in this population.

10. C. Point estimation and confidence interval are tools used for estimating population values based on samples, and they are not related to hypothesis testing.

SUGGESTED READING

Altman, D.G., 1980. Statistics and ethics in medical research: III How large a sample? Br Med J 281, 1336–1338.

Basic statistics for clinicians, 1995. Can. Med. Assoc. J. <www.cmaj.ca>.

Centre for Evidence Based Medicine, Department of Medicine, Toronto General Hospital, Toronto. <www.cebm.utoronto.ca>.

Drummond, J.P., Silva, E., 1998. Medicina Baseada em Evidências: Novo Paradigma Assistencial e Pedagógico. Atheneu, Sao Paulo, Brazil.

Estrela, C., 2001. Metodologia Científica Ensino e Pesquisa em Odontologia. Editora Artes Médicas, Sao Paulo, Brazil.

Everitt, B., 2006. Medical Statistics from A to Z: A Guide for Clinicians and Medical Students, second ed. Cambridge University Press, Cambridge, UK.

Everitt, B.S., 1995. The Cambridge Dictionary of Statistics in the Medical Sciences. Cambridge University Press, Cambridge, UK.

Everitt, B.S., et al., 2005. Encyclopaedic Companion to Medical Statistics. Hodder Arnold, London.

Hulley, S.B., et al., 2001. Designing Clinical Research: An Epidemiological Approach, second ed. Lippincott Williams & Wilkins, Philadelphia.

Merriam–Webster Online Dictionary. <www.merriam-webster.com>.

Microsoft Excel Glossary. <www.intelligentedu.com/microsoft_excel_glossary.html>.

Neto, P.L.O.C., 1977. Estatística. Editora Edgard Blücher, Sao Paulo, Brazil.

Oliveira, G.G., 2006. Ensaios Clínicos Princípios e Prática. Editora Anvisa, Brasília, Brazil.

Sackett, D.L., et al., 2001. Evidence-Based Medicine: How to Practice and Teach EBM, second ed. Churchill Livingstone, Edinburgh, UK.

Schmuller, J., 2009. Statistical Analysis with Excel for Dummies, second ed. Wiley, Hoboken, NJ.

Whitley, E., Ball, J., 2002. Statistics review 4: Sample size calculations. Crit Care 6, 335–341.

Additional Concepts in Biostatistics

The objective of Part IV is to expand the reader's proficiency by dissertating on other statistical approaches adopted in clinical research. The chapters were developed independently, and they can be studied separately.

Chapter 11

Individual and Collective Benefit and Risk Indexes Inferable from Intervention Studies

In addition to statistical significance (p) and 95% confidence interval, it is feasible to extend the usefulness of data collected from a clinical study through collective, as well as individual, benefit and risk indexes. Such indexes are especially useful tools in the clinical setting.

In order to demonstrate these concepts, we adopt here an example based on a clinical trial: subcutaneous ondaparin for the prevention of venous thromboembolism in intensive care unit admitted medical patients in a randomized, placebo-controlled trial ($n = 644$ patients (ondaparin, 321 patients; placebo, 323 patients)). From its results, we can tabulate undesired event (deep venous thrombosis (DVT)) and adverse reactions rates associated with the tested therapy (Tables 11.1 and 11.2, respectively). Some hypothetical rates are also useful to further detail additional concepts. The following acronyms are used:

UEC: undesired event rate in the control group
UEE: undesired event rate in the experimental group
ARC: adverse reaction rate in the control group
ARE: adverse reaction rate in the experimental group

Several indexes may be inferred from Tables 11.1 and 11.2, and these are discussed next.

11.1 TREATMENT EFFECT INDEXES

Treatment effect indexes refer to expected collective occurrence rates and are not applicable in the setting of individual patients.

11.1.1 Risk Indexes

The risk indexes to be detailed here are the basal, relative, relative risk reduction, absolute risk reduction, relative risk increase, absolute risk increase and odds ratio.

M. Suchmacher & M. Geller: Practical Biostatistics. DOI: 10.1016/B978-0-12-415794-1.00011-2

TABLE 11.1 Undesired Event Rates (DVT) from Ondaparin Clinical Trial

	UEC (%)	UEE (%)
Undesired event real rate	10.5	5.6
Undesired event hypothetical rate	20	4
Extremely low undesired event hypothetical rate	0.1	0.05
Extremely high undesired event hypothetical rate	95	90

TABLE 11.2 Adverse Reaction Rates from Ondaparin Trial[a]

	Adverse Reaction Rate (%)
ARC	1.2
ARE	3.2

[a]Some data have been changed for didactic purposes.

Basal Risk

Basal risk (BR) refers to the degree of risk in the control group with regard to undesired events as well as adverse reactions (in our example, 10.5 and 3.2%, respectively).

Relative Risk

Relative risk (RR) determines the degree of risk for the undesired event in the subgroup that presented it (experimental group) relative to BR (Figure 11.1). It is calculated by the following formula:

$$\frac{UEE \times 100}{UEC}$$

$$\frac{5.6 \times 100}{10.5} = 53\%$$

The previous result means that the subgroup that presented the undesired event (experimental group) had a degree of risk of 53% relative to the opposite corresponding subgroup (control group). In other words, if the patients of the subgroup that presented the undesired event (control group) had received ondaparin, only 53% of them would have presented DVT.

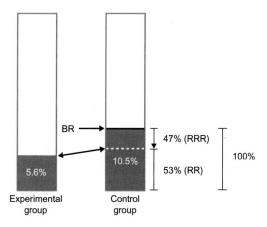

FIGURE 11.1   Schematic representation of relative risk.

This index is limited by a reduction in its capacity to express valid results whenever extremely low or high frequencies are reported (Table 11.1):

- RR calculated for extremely low hypothetical rates

$$\frac{0.05 \times 100}{0.1} = 50\%$$

Although the number of patients represented by these hypothetical frequencies is neglectful (0.3 patients on placebo and 0.1 patients on ondaparin), relative risk reduction would be relatively high. Ondaparin association with a decrease in DVT frequency would therefore be overestimated. In this setting, odds ratio (see Section 1.1.7) would be a more suitable index.

- RR calculated for extremely high hypothetical rates (Figure 11.2)

$$\frac{90 \times 100}{95} = 95\%$$

The important difference between the number of patients in the subgroup that presented DVT (control group) relative to the opposite corresponding subgroup (experimental group) (307 − 289 = 18 patients) would point to a considerable ondaparin efficacy. However, a 95% RR suggests that this efficacy would nevertheless be exaggerated.

Relative Risk Reduction

Relative risk reduction (RRR) determines the degree of risk reduction for the undesired event in the subgroup that presented it (experimental group) relative to the opposite corresponding subgroup (control group). It is calculated by the following formula:

$$\frac{UEE - UEC}{UEC}$$

$$\frac{5.6 - 10.5}{10.5} = -0.46 \text{ (or 46\%)}$$

Observe the histogram shown in Figure 11.1.

The previous result means that ondaparin was associated with a 46% DVT risk reduction in the subgroup that presented this undesired event (experimental group) relative to the opposite corresponding subgroup (control group). In other words, if the patients of the subgroup that presented the undesired event (control group) had received ondaparin, they would have had a 46% less probability of presenting DVT.

Similar to RR, RRR is limited by a reduction in its capacity to express valid results whenever extremely low or high frequencies are reported (Table 11.1):

- RRR calculated for extremely low hypothetical rates

$$\frac{0.05 - 0.1}{0.1} = -0.5 \text{ (or 50\%)}$$

Although the number of patients represented by these hypothetical frequencies is insignificant (0.006 patients on placebo and 0.003 patients on fondparinux), RRR reached 50%. The association of ondaparin with DVT frequency decrease was therefore overestimated. In this setting, odds ratio (see Section 11.1.1) would be a more suitable index.

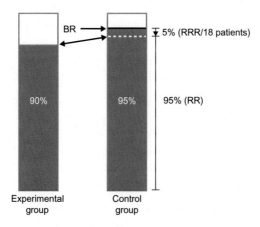

FIGURE 11.2   Schematic representation of relative risk in an extremely high hypothetical rates setting.

- RRR calculated for extremely high hypothetical rates (observe the histogram shown in Figure 11.2)

$$\frac{90 - 95}{95} = -0.05 \text{ (or 5\%)}$$

The important difference between the number of patients in the subgroup that presented DVT (control group) relative to the opposite corresponding subgroup (experimental group) ($307 - 289 = 18$ patients) would point to a considerable ondaparin efficacy. However, RRR was only 5%. Ondaparin efficacy in decreasing DVT frequency was therefore underestimated.

Absolute Risk Reduction

Absolute risk reduction (ARR) determines the degree of risk reduction for the undesired event between control (BR) and experimental groups (Figure 11.3). It is calculated by the simple arithmetic difference between UEC and UEE:

$$10.5 - 5.6 \cong 5\%$$

The previous result means that if ondaparin had been used in all of the patients in the control group, they would have had a 5% less probability of presenting DVT.

The following are differences between ARR and RRR:

- Greater proximity to "real world" scenarios
  Whereas RRR focuses only on the subgroups that presented the undesired event, ARR encompasses the whole group (the subgroup that

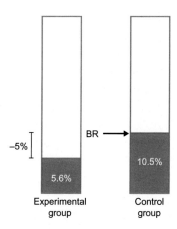

FIGURE 11.3   Schematic representation of absolute risk reduction.

presented and the subgroup that did not present the undesired event, from both groups). This assumption takes into consideration not only the risk variability among those who presented the undesired event but also BR variability. This is a situation that more closely reflects the decision-making processes in the "real world" because one cannot know beforehand if a procedure might direct a patient either to the subgroup that will present or to the subgroup that will not present the undesired event.

- Protection against distorted results based on extremely low values

    Observe ARR calculated for extremely low hypothetical rates (Table 11.1):

$$0.1 - 0.05 \cong 0.05\%$$

It is obvious that there is no significant ARR in the previous example, even though the corresponding RRR (see RRR calculated for extremely low hypothetical rates) suggests the opposite.

A 5% RRR index based on real rates is consistent with what is inferable from a 46% RRR − that is, that there is a risk reduction in DVT among older medical patients under ondaparin relative to placebo. Therefore, one can consider the possibility of spurious interpretations due to mathematical nuances as unlikely.

One ARR limitation is its decreased capacity of BR variability expression in situations in which RR and RRR variability prevail, along with a constant ARR. Observe the hypothetical evolving example detailed in Figure 11.4. RRR and RR clearly better expressed evolutive BR variability than did ARR, which remained equal (10%) from Time 1 to Time 2.

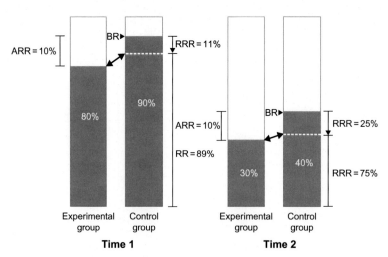

FIGURE 11.4   Schematic representation of an evolving sample (Time 1 and Time 2), where BR seems to express different meanings.

Relative Risk Increase

Relative risk increase (RRI) determines the degree of risk increase for an adverse reaction in the subgroup that presented it (experimental group) relative to the opposite corresponding subgroup (control group). It is calculated by the following formula:

$$\frac{UEE - UEC}{UEC}$$

$$\frac{3.2 - 1.2}{1.2} = 1.6 \text{ (or } +60\%)$$

The previous result means that if ondaparin had been used in all patients in the subgroup that presented hemorrhage (control group), they would have had a 60% greater probability of presenting this adverse reaction.

Absolute Risk Increase

Absolute risk increase (ARI) determines the degree of risk increase for an adverse reaction in an experimental group. It is calculated by the simple arithmetic difference between ARE and ARC:

$$3.2 - 1.2 = 2.0\%$$

The previous result means that if ondaparin had been used in all patients in the control group, they would have had a 2% greater probability of presenting hemorrhage episodes.

Whereas RRI focuses only on the subgroups that presented the adverse reaction, ARI encompasses the whole group (the subgroup that presented and the subgroup that did not present the adverse reaction, from both groups). This assumption takes into consideration not only the risk variability among those who presented the adverse reaction but also BR variability. This is a situation that more closely reflects decision-making processes in the "real world" because one cannot know beforehand if a procedure might direct a patient to either the subgroup that will present or the subgroup that will not present the adverse reaction.

Odds Ratio

In the clinical trial setting, odds ratio (OR) expresses the odds for the occurrence of an undesired event in the experimental group relative to the same odds in the control group. Let us calculate the ratio between the undesired event odds in the ondaparin group and the same odds in the placebo group:

$$\frac{UEE/(100 - UEE)}{UEC/(100 - UEC)} = \frac{0.06}{0.12} = 0.5$$

The previous result means that the experimental group had a 0.5:1 ratio of presenting an undesired event relative to the control group. OR expresses essentially the same as RR, with the following differences:

- Internists and surgeons expect to obtain immediate applicable information from intervention studies, and the type of information detailed here is often better captured in the practice setting as risk rather than as odds: To inform that ondaparin affords a 53% reduction in DVT risk is generally better understood than stating that ondaparin presents a 0.5:1 odds for this undesired event.
- RR informs more clearly on no treatment effect than does OR: Not administering ondaparin would increase DVT risk in 47% $(100 - 53\%)$ of patients.
- OR informs on the undesired event occurrence odds in the groups as a whole, which is more appealing information in the epidemiological setting, whereas RR focuses on how much BR is prone to variation between subgroups, which is more relevant information in the practice setting.
- OR is a more suitable resource to estimate degree of association between an exposure factor and risk of an undesired event for low rate events.

OR presents greater usefulness in case—control observational studies (Chapters 1 and 3) and in meta-analyses (Chapter 4).

11.1.2 Benefit Indexes

The benefit indexes to be detailed here are absolute benefit increase and relative benefit increase.

Absolute Benefit Increase

Absolute benefit increase determines the degree of benefit increase in the experimental group (where benefit is defined as the non-occurrence of the undesired event). It is calculated by the simple arithmetic difference between the rate of the benefited subgroup (control group) and the rate of the opposite corresponding subgroup (experimental group):

$$94.4 - 89.5 \simeq 5\%$$

The previous result means that ondaparin use by the experimental group was associated with a 5% probability increase for this group of not presenting DVT.

Relative Benefit Increase

Relative benefit increase determines the degree of benefit increase in the benefited subgroup (experimental group) relative to the opposite corresponding subgroup (control group) (where benefit is defined as the non-occurrence of the undesired event):

$$\frac{94.4 - 89.5}{89.5} = 0.05 \text{ (or 5\%)}$$

The previous result means that ondaparin use by the benefited subgroup (experimental group) was associated with a 5% probability for this subgroup of not presenting DVT relative to the opposite corresponding subgroup.

11.1.3 Number Needed to Treat

Number needed to treat (NNT) corresponds to the number of individuals who must be treated so that one subject benefits from the treatment. It is calculated by the following formula:

$$\frac{1}{\text{ARR}}$$

$$\frac{1}{5^*} = 0.20 = 20$$

The previous result means that if ondaparin had been used in the control group, it would have been necessary to treat 20 patients so that 1 patient would not present DVT. It corresponds to ARR, expressed in a different manner.

Obviously, changes in the elements that determine ARR − UEE and UEC − will influence NNT. As a general rule, NNT changes inversely with BR; that is, the higher the BR (and therefore UEC), the lower NNT is expected to be. Observe NNT calculated for undesired event hypothetical rate (Table 11.1):

$$\frac{1}{20 - 4}$$

$$\frac{1}{16} = 0.06 = 6$$

A greater ARR difference (16 to 5%*) might represent a greater therapeutic efficacy in terms of undesired event avoidance. As such, a smaller number of patients to treat would be necessary so that one of them would benefit. It is inferable that ondaparin administration would be more advantageous in the latter situation than in the former.

The main use for NNT is to make ARR data more practical to physicians and comprehensible to patients. Its interpretation must be performed based on the physician's own practice experience and on NNTs established for other treatment modalities related to the case. NNT is not as statistically as sound as ARR.

The following are additional NNT examples:

- Intensive insulin regimen for 6.5 years for diabetic neuropathy prevention: 15 patients
- Streptokinase administration followed by daily aspirin for 5 weeks for acute myocardial infarction death prevention: 29 patients
- Anti-hypertensive medication for 5.5 years for acute myocardial infarction, stroke, and death prevention: 128 patients

11.1.4 Number Needed to Harm

Number needed to harm (NNH) corresponds to the number of individuals who must be treated so that one of them presents an adverse reaction accountable to the treatment. It is calculated by the following formula:

$$\frac{1}{ARI}$$

$$\frac{1}{2} = 0.5 = 50$$

The previous result means that if the control group had used ondaparin, it would have been necessary to treat 50 patients so that 1 patient would not present an adverse reaction accountable to the treatment. It corresponds to ARI, expressed in a different manner.

The main use for NNH is to make ARI data more practical to physicians and comprehensible to patients. Its interpretation must be performed based on the physician's own practice experience and on NNHs established for other treatment modalities related to the case.

11.1.5 Likelihood of Being Helped Versus Being Harmed

Likelihood of being helped versus being harmed (LLH) is an aggregation ratio that takes NNT and NNH into account:

$$\frac{1}{NNT} : \frac{1}{NNH}$$

$$\frac{1}{20} : \frac{1}{50} \Rightarrow 3 : 1$$

The previous result means that ondaparin treatment has a probability of 3 of benefiting study patients compared to a probability of 1 of harming them.

11.2 CLINICAL DECISION ANALYSIS INDEXES

Clinical decision analysis indexes refer to expected occurrence rates related to a specific patient in the practice setting based on results of clinical studies or empirical estimatives. Assuming that in the practice setting one must take into consideration the potential benefits as well as the potential risks of a treatment modality, these indexes shall take both into account. There are three ways of expressing this type of information.

11.2.1 Patient-Specific Number Needed to Treat

Suppose it is necessary to know NNT for a specific patient in such a way that the least possible degree of risk is expected from the considered therapeutic modality. This index can be calculated by two formulas:

- $$\frac{1}{PEER \times RRR}$$

where PEER is the patient expected event rate, and RRR is the relative risk reduction.

PEER and RRR may be taken from literary sources that describe a control group consistent with the specific patient. By applying the ondaparin study as an example (with PEER corresponding to UEC; Table 11.1), we obtain the following:

$$\frac{1}{10.5 \times 46} = 0.002 = 20$$

The previous result means that it would be necessary to treat 20 patients in the same way as the specific patient in order to obtain a positive result, expecting the least possible degree of risk.

- $$\frac{NNT}{f_t}$$

NNT may be taken from literary sources (e.g. the ondaparin study); f_t (fraction$_{treatment}$) may be taken from two sources:

- Empirical estimatives

    One estimates that the specific patient, if left untreated, would have twice the risk of presenting the undesired event relative to that of a treated patient.

- Literary sources that present control and experimental groups consistent with the case of the specific patient

    In the ondaparin study, patients from the subgroup that presented the undesired event (control group) showed twice the risk for DVT relative to patients from the opposite corresponding subgroup (experimental group):

$$\frac{20}{2} = 10$$

The previous result means that it would be necessary to treat 10 patients in the same way as the specific patient in order to obtain a positive result, expecting the least possible degree of risk.

Both formulas for patient-specific NNT determination express essentially the same information. The differences are that (1) the latter is easier to apply, and (2) it allows us to use data obtained from our own clinical experience.

11.2.2 Patient-Specific Number Needed to Harm

Suppose we are seeing an individual patient who we deem is especially susceptible to a therapeutic adverse reaction, and we want to more precisely identify the risks that he or she is about to take. This index can be calculated by the following formula:

$$\frac{\text{NNH}}{f_h}$$

NNH may be taken from literary sources (e.g. the ondaparin study); f_h (fraction$_{harm}$) may be taken from two sources:

- Empirical estimative

    One estimates that a patient such as ours has a twofold risk of presenting the adverse reaction relative to a nontreated patient:

$$\frac{50}{2} = 25$$

- RRI from literary sources consistent with our patient's case (e.g. the ondaparin study):

$$\frac{50}{1.6} = 31$$

The previous result means that it would be necessary to treat 25 (or 31) patients like ours so that one of them would present an adverse reaction accountable to the treatment.

11.2.3 Patient-Specific Likelihood of Being Helped Versus Being Harmed

Patient-specific LHH is an index that expresses the same information detailed in Section 11.1.5, adjusted for a specific patient. It is calculated by the following ratio:

$$(1/\text{NNT} \times f_t) : (1/\text{NNH} \times f_h)$$
$$(0.05 \times 2) : (0.02 \times 1.6) \Rightarrow 3 : 1$$

The previous result means that ondaparin treatment has a probability of 3 of benefiting the specific patient compared to a probability of 1 of harming him or her.

Chapter 12

Statistical Assessment of Diagnostic Tests for the Clinic

An investigator may perform a study to test a new exam or diagnostic procedure. Similarly, a health professional may face the decision of which diagnostic test should be used for a specific patient, what to expect from it, and how to interpret the available literature to support his or her conduct. In the diagnostic test setting, this approach can be performed with the aid of specific mathematical tools. We discuss this concept using a practical example:

Suppose you see a patient in the emergency room who complains of precordial pain that started less than 6 hours ago. An electrocardiogram (ECG) is performed, and the results are inconclusive for acute coronary failure. Your institution has a nuclear medicine facility in which single-photon emission computed tomography (SPECT) can be performed in order to document the perfusional deficit (if there is any). However, before ordering the test, you want to gather more evidence that it might be useful for your patient.

You search the literature and find a clinical trial consistent with your case: myocardial perfusion scintigraphy (SPECT) in the evaluation of emergency room patients with precordial pain and normal or doubtful ischemic ECG. The study includes 60 cases. You move to the next step, which is to determine indexes of disease detection capacity and diagnostic significance of the considered test based on the trial data, the results of which are detailed in Table 12.1. Based on these data, the usefulness of the test can be determined by the indexes discussed in the following sections

12.1 DETECTION CAPACITY INDEXES

Detection capacity indexes determine a test capacity for detecting individuals with a condition and for not detecting those individuals who do not have it.

M. Suchmacher & M. Geller: Practical Biostatistics. DOI: 10.1016/B978-0-12-415794-1.00012-4
153

TABLE 12.1 Results from SPECT in a Coronary Failure Trial[a]

	Patients with Coronary Failure	Patients without Coronary Failure	Total
Altered scintigraphy	19 (a)	10 (b)	29
Normal scintigraphy	6 (c)	25 (d)	31
Total	25	35	60

[a]Some data were changed for didactic purposes.

12.1.1 Sensitivity

Sensitivity determines the capacity of a test to detect individuals with a condition from a population in which all individuals have it. It is calculated by the following formula:

$$a/(a+c)$$
$$19/(19+6) = 0.76 = 76\%$$

The previous result means that SPECT has a 76% probability of detecting coronary failure in an individual who actually has it. The higher this proportion, the lower the probability of a false-negative yield, and the greater the probability for condition nonexistence in the case of a negative yield.

12.1.2 Specificity

Specificity determines the capacity of a test to not detect an altered test result in a population whose individuals do not have the considered condition. It is calculated by the following formula:

$$d/(b+d)$$
$$25/(10+25) = 0.71 = 71\%$$

The previous result means that SPECT has a 71% probability of not detecting coronary failure in an individual who actually does not have it. By inference, it has a 29% probability of detecting this condition in an individual who does not have it. The greater the sensitivity, the lower the probability of a false-positive result, and the greater the probability for condition existence in the case of a positive result.

12.1.3 Likelihood Ratio

Likelihood ratio (LR) is an index that aggregates sensitivity and specificity, strengthening conclusions inferable from both. It is expressed in two ways.

Positive Likelihood Ratio

Positive LR determines the probability of a test in detecting condition A instead of condition B, which could also change test results. It is calculated by the following formula:

$$\text{Sensitivity}/(100 - \text{specificity})$$
$$76\%/(100\% - 71\%) = 2.6$$

The previous result means that SPECT has a 2.6 greater probability of detecting coronary failure than other causes potentially associated with an altered SPECT result, such as myocarditis.

As a general rule, the following ranges for LR result interpretation can be adopted:

>10: The test has a high capacity for detecting the suspected condition.
~1: The test has a limited capacity for detecting the suspected condition.
<0.1: The test has a low capacity for detecting the suspected condition.

Negative Likelihood Ratio

Negative LR determines the probability of a test in detecting condition B, which could also change test results, instead of condition A. It is calculated by the following formula:

$$(100 - \text{sensitivity})/\text{specificity}$$
$$(100 - 76)/71 = 0.33$$

The previous result means that SPECT has a 0.33 greater probability of detecting a condition other than coronary failure, rather than coronary failure itself.

According to these detection capacity indexes, SPECT has a good capacity for coronary failure detection in a patient with less than 6 hours precordial pain and a doubtful ECG.

12.2 DIAGNOSTIC SIGNIFICANCE INDEXES

Diagnostic significance indexes determine the capacity of a positive test result in representing a condition existence and of a negative yield in not representing it.

12.2.1 Pretest Probability (Prevalence)

Pretest probability determines the proportion of individuals with a condition in relation to a population under risk. It is calculated by the following formula:

$$(a + c)/(a + b + c + d)$$
$$25/60 = 0.41 = 41\%$$

Pretest probability is useful for pretest odds calculation.

12.2.2 Pretest Odds

Pretest odds determine the odds of an individual belonging to a population at risk of presenting a condition. The higher the prevalence, the higher the odds. They are calculated by the following formula:

$$\text{Prevalence}/(1 - \text{prevalence})$$
$$0.41/0.59 = 0.69$$

Results range from 0 (null odds) to 1.0 (the highest possible odds). Pretest odds are useful in post-test odds calculation.

12.2.3 Post-Test Odds

Post-test odds determine the odds of an individual who presents a positive test result of actually having the suspected condition. They are calculated by the following formula:

$$\text{Pretest odds} \times \text{positive likelihood ratio}$$
$$0.69 \times 2.6 = 1.8$$

The previous result represents a 1.8:1 post-test odds for the actual presence of coronary failure in an individual with a positive SPECT.

12.2.4 Post-Test Probability

Post-test probability determines the proportion of individuals presenting a positive test result who actually have the suspected condition. It is calculated by the following formula:

$$\text{Post-test odds}/(\text{post-test odds} + 1)$$
$$1.8/2.8 = 0.64 = 64\%$$

Post-test probability expresses essentially the same results as post-test odds but from a collective perspective.

12.2.5 Positive Predictive Value

Positive predictive value determines the proportion of individuals presenting a positive test result who actually have the suspected condition. It is calculated by the following formula:

$$a/(a + b)$$
$$19/29 = 0.65 = 65\%$$

Positive predictive value expresses essentially the same result as post-test probability, but it does so through a different mathematical approach.

12.2.6 Negative Predictive Value

Negative predictive value determines the proportion of individuals presenting a negative test result who actually do not have the suspected condition. It is calculated by the following formula:

$$d/(c + d)$$
$$25/31 = 0.80 = 80\%$$

It expresses the probability of a test in not yielding a false-positive result.

Based on the overall results presented previously, one can infer that a positive myocardial perfusion scintigraphy (SPECT) test indicates a good probability for coronary failure in a patient with precordial pain complaint lasting less than 6 hours, and an ECG inconclusive for ischemic heart disease.

The determination of the prevalence of a condition is essential for calculation of post-test odds/post-test probability indexes. An available source from which this information could be extracted was used in the previous examples (a clinical trial involving the investigated procedure). However, different sources can be explored if no immediate consistent studies are available:

- Personal or institutional data bank
  - For example, your hospital records show that 34 patients are diagnosed with coronary failure out of every 100 patients admitted to the emergency room.
- Statistical database from public health institutions
- Scientific studies of prevalence determination of several different conditions

However, because it is likely that data from different sources will be mathematically gathered, it is advisable to ask for the support of a biostatistician.

The following are examples of detection capacity and diagnostic significance indexes already published:

- Serum ferritin determination for iron deficiency anemia diagnosis
  - Sensitivity: 90.4%
  - Specificity: 84.7%
  - Positive predictive value: 73%
  - Negative predictive value: 95%
  - Post-test odds: 2.6
- D-dimer serum levels greater than 1092 mg/mL for deep venous thrombosis detection in inpatients with stroke sequelae: LR 3.1
- Manual device-determined serum heart-specific troponin T levels for myocardial infarction detection within 2 hours of clinical onset:
  - LR+ : 6.3
  - LR− : 0.8

Chapter 13

Systematic Reviews and Meta-Analyses

13.1 DEFINITIONS

- Systematic review: Comprehensive, protocol-based, and reproducible bibliographic review of randomized clinical trials (primary studies). It aims to test a clearly stated investigator's hypothesis and is a preceding stage to a meta-analysis.
- Meta-analysis: A statistical procedure that aims to determine efficacy or nonefficacy, generally of a medical intervention, through analysis of data across primary studies selected by systematic review in order to generate an average pooled estimate of their effect sizes. In principle, meta-analyses afford a more powerful statistical testing than respective primary studies separately.

Meta-analyses can include the following endpoints:

- Relative risk, odds ratio, absolute risk reduction, and number needed to treat (Chapter 11)
- Scores
- Sensitivity and specificity (Chapter 12)
- p values (Chapter 4)

13.2 SYSTEMATIC REVIEW

Systematic reviews can be performed in three stages.

13.2.1 Problem Formulation

Investigator's hypothesis (Chapter 4) must be explicitly formulated, as for any other scientific study.

13.2.2 Primary Studies Search and Selection

This stage is performed by a member of the research team called the "searcher." The following are proposed guidelines:

- Search criteria and determination of minimum quality level of primary studies must be stated in the study protocol:
  - Are primary studies randomized?

M. Suchmacher & M. Geller: Practical Biostatistics. DOI: 10.1016/B978-0-12-415794-1.00013-6

- Was the studied object compared to an adequate control?
- Were there adjustments for eventual differences among elements of the several primary studies?
- Was the studied sample representative of the target population, quantitatively as well as qualitatively?
- Were study subjects sufficiently homogeneous with regard to prognosis?

- Primary studies must be cross-consistent regarding the following aspects:
  - Population type
  - Type of condition
  - Type of intervention
  - Methodology
  - Type of outcome
- Search results must be reproduced by an independent reviewer, and this reproduction must be statistically validated.
- Language restrictions must be avoided.
- Non-normal distribution studies (Chapter 6) must be ruled out.
- Search must be thorough, and every possible source must be considered: databases, sponsoring agencies, studies of pharmaceutical companies, regulatory agencies, post-graduation dissertations and theses, and clinical trial registries.

Discrepancies between searcher and independent reviewer findings can be resolved through statistical methodology or by a second independent reviewer.

13.2.3 Primary Studies Data Extraction

The searcher's objective in this stage is to organize extracted data from primary studies in order to determine if meta-analysis is feasible. Its methodology is based on the following guidelines:

- Performed according to a specially designed form.
- Search results must be reproduced by an independent reviewer.
- Extraction should be "blind"; that is, the name of the authors of primary studies must be concealed.
- The data extraction process can be extended through direct contact with the authors of primary studies (this procedure would obviously nullify the "blindness" status of the research, and this should be stated).
- Extracted data must be tabulated for insertion in a suitable software.

Discrepancies between searcher and independent reviewer findings can be resolved through statistical methodology or by a second independent reviewer.

13.3 META-ANALYSIS

A meta-analysis is not merely an arithmetic mean of the results from the different primary studies but, rather, an elaborate methodology that aims to determine the weighted mean of effect sizes of pooled primary studies selected from a systematic review. Meta-analysis can be performed in four stages.

13.3.1 Publication Bias Detection

Publication bias can be investigated with the aid of a funnel plot graph (Figure 13.1). The weighted mean of effect sizes (pooled estimate of effects) (see Section 13.3.4) corresponds to the funnel axis. The larger the n of a primary study, the larger its corresponding weight in a pooled estimate of effects determination. This is the reason why corresponding blocks tend to stand closer to the funnel axis. The opposite is true for primary studies with a smaller n due to their larger results variability.

This type of distribution tends to generate a characteristic funnel-shaped plotting. Publication bias can be visualized through graphic paucity of primary studies (trapezoid field), which are generally associated with negative results and/or a small n. As such, the closer the funnel plot is to a pyramid shape, the weaker the publication bias. Publication bias level and the extent to which it compromises meta-analysis quality must be determined by the investigators.

13.3.2 Heterogeneity Analysis

Primary studies heterogeneity caused by between-study differences is an expected circumstance. Its analysis is crucial for defining whether selected primary studies pooling is fit for meta-analysis. Heterogeneity can manifest in two ways, with corresponding procedures:

- Clinical heterogeneity: It requires assessment based on clinical grounds.

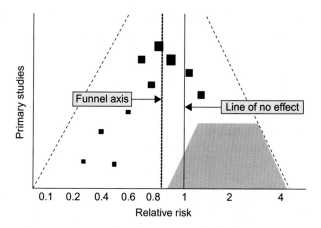

FIGURE 13.1 Main landmarks of a funnel plot graph.

- Methodological heterogeneity: It requires statistical quantification. In this case, null hypothesis (Chapter 4) assumes that primary studies are heterogeneous among themselves. Therefore, rejecting H_0 means that there is sufficient homogeneity ($p < 0.10$ is generally acceptable) among these studies. The limitation of statistical tests is that their power to detect statistically significant homogeneity is weakened among primary studies with a small n and with pools of few primary studies.

If homogeneity is not demonstrated, it is not advisable to upgrade the systematic review to meta-analysis.

13.3.3 Summarized Statistical Determination

Summarized statistical determination corresponds to effect size specification of each individual primary study. It is a necessary step for meta-analysis weighted mean determination.

13.3.4 Meta-Analysis Performance and Expression

Pooled estimate of individual effect sizes of primary studies can be calculated as a weighted mean:

$$\text{Meta-analysis weighted mean} = \frac{\sum T_i W_i}{\sum W_i}$$

where i is the individual study, T_i is the effect size attributed to i primary study, and W_i is the weight attributed to i primary study.

Standard error of the mean (Chapter 6) of this pooled estimate can be used to determine 95% confidence interval (Chapter 10) and corresponding p.

One of the most popular ways of graphically representing meta-analysis results is the use of a forest plot (confidence intervals plotting). Its graphical elements are depicted in Figure 13.2.

- Block: The block represents the weighted mean (point estimate) of primary study x. Its relative size and proximity to the meta-analysis pooled estimate (meta-analysis weighted mean) are proportional to primary study x relative weight.
- 95% confidence interval line: The 95% confidence interval line represents the primary study x confidence interval. The narrower it is, the larger primary study x weight and proximity to meta-analysis pooled estimate are expected to be. In order to be significant for meta-analysis, it must not touch the "line of no effect."
- Significance line (line of no effect): The significance line represents outcome variable value neutrality.
- Meta-analysis weighted mean: The meta-analysis weighted mean vertically represents the weighted mean of effect sizes, obtained by meta-analysis.

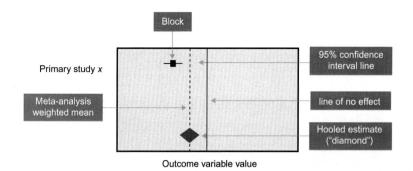

FIGURE 13.2   Main landmarks of a forest plot graph.

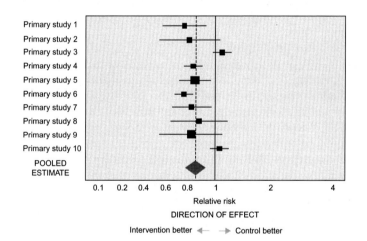

FIGURE 13.3   Result of a meta-analysis on the efficacy of a vaccine, expressed as a forest plot.

- Pooled estimate: The pooled estimate represents the weighted mean of effect sizes, obtained by meta-analysis. Its width corresponds to its 95% confidence interval.

An example of a hypothetical meta-analysis on the efficacy of a vaccine is shown in Figure 13.3. A pooled estimate demonstrates a protective effect provided by the vaccine. Nevertheless, the statistical significance of this result must also be determined.

The following are additional data for the forest plot:

- *n*
- Mean with standard deviation
- *p* of each primary study

- Meta-analysis overall 95% confidence interval
- Heterogeneity test result, with statistical significance

Meta-analysis statistical significance level, p, must also be established.

13.4 OPTIONS IF META-ANALYSIS PERFORMANCE IS NOT ADVISABLE

- Keep the research as systematic review only.
- Perform a subgroup meta-analysis.

    In a subgroup meta-analysis, a heterogeneous population of primary studies is subdivided into two homogeneous subgroups. The result can be expressed as a forest plot graph. A meta-analysis involving 10 primary studies considered as heterogeneous is exemplified in Figure 13.4. Two separate pooled estimates are obtainable by dividing the different primary studies in subgroups (Figure 13.5).

- Perform sensitivity analysis.

    Sensitivity analysis consists of a re-analysis of the data set of primary studies, aiming to determine if identifying possible confounders (type of intervention, subject profile, and outcome variables) or decreasing heterogeneity among them could lead to a different final outcome or interpretation. This procedure might allow a new meta-analysis trial.

- Perform meta-regression analysis.

    Meta-regression analysis is a statistical procedure that aims to identify and quantify sources of heterogeneity among primary studies. Tools such as multiple linear regression (Chapter 14) or logistic regression are employed in order to explore the relationship among the parameters of primary studies, such as geographical location, subjects' age, and effect size.

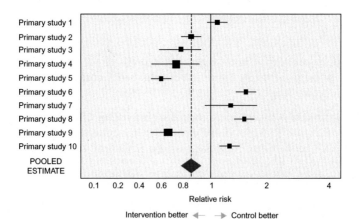

FIGURE 13.4   Result of a meta-analysis on 10 heterogeneous primary studies.

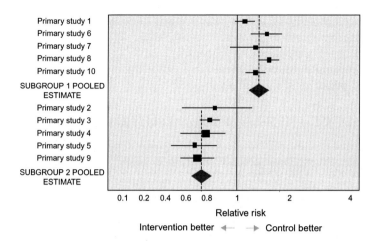

FIGURE 13.5 Result of a subgroup meta-analysis after division of primary studies as subgroups.

13.5 SYSTEMATIC REVIEW/META-ANALYSIS LIMITATIONS

- Publication bias
  - Positive studies are more likely to be published.
  - Primary studies are more likely to be published in English.
  - Positive studies are published more swiftly than negative studies.
  - Larger n studies are more likely to be published.
  - Smaller n studies are more likely to be published if they present positive results.
- Searcher and independent reviewer learning curve
  - Inexperienced searchers and independent reviewers tend to make assessment and methodological errors during the research. Participation of an experienced researcher may compensate for this limitation.

13.6 SYSTEMATIC REVIEW/META-ANALYSIS STAGES SUMMARY

- Systematic review
  - Problem formulation
  - Primary studies search and selection
  - Primary studies data extraction
- Meta-analysis
  - Publication bias detection
  - Heterogeneity analysis
  - Summarized statistics determination
  - Meta-analysis performance and expression

- Options if meta-analysis performance is not advisable
  - Keep research as systematic review only
  - Perform subgroup meta-analysis
  - Perform sensitivity analysis
  - Perform meta-regression analysis

13.7 SUGGESTED RESOURCES AND LITERARY SOURCES

- PubMed (Medline) (free access): www.pubmed.gov
- Embase (subscription access): www.embase.com
- Cochrane Controlled Trials Register (CENTRAL): www.cochrane.org
- NLM Gateway (free access): gateway.nlm.nih.gov
- LILACS (Latin America and the Caribbean Literature on Health Sciences) (free access): lilacs.bvsalud.org (English language link available on the homepage)
- DARE (Database of Abstracts of Reviews of Effects; Centre for Reviews and Dissemination, York University) (free access): www.crd.york.ac.uk/cms2web
- EndNote (bibliographic management software): www.endnote.com
- RevMan (Cochrane group reviews software): ims.cochrane.org/RevMan
- Comprehensive Meta-Analysis (software): www.meta-analysis.com

Chapter 14

Correlation and Regression

Sometimes, the investigator's hypothesis does not involve searching for statistically significant differences between groups but, rather, how well two different study variables relate to each other. If they do significantly relate to each other, then predicting the value of one variable based on the value of the other one may be feasible. Two mathematical tools are available to accomplish these objectives: correlation and regression.

14.1 CORRELATION

Correlation has two goals: (1) to quantify the degree of connection between a pair of variables and (2) to determine the direction of this relationship. Biological plausibility demands that, in the clinical setting, the "strongest" variable influences the "more susceptible" one. This proposition implies two opposing concepts:

- Independent variable: The independent variable is the variable that has influence on the dependent variable but in turn is not influenced by the latter. In didactic terms, it is the "dominant" variable. For example, body temperature (independent variable) influences heart rate (dependent variable) rather than the opposite. By convention, it is identified as x and graphically represented by the horizontal axis (x-axis).
- Dependent variable: The dependent variable is the variable that is influenced by the independent variable but in turn has no influence on the latter. In didactic terms, it is the "submissive" variable. For example, heart rate (dependent variable) is influenced by body temperature (independent variable) rather than the opposite. By convention, it is identified as y and graphically represented by the vertical axis (y-axis).

Take, for example, a cohort of 26 overweight middle-aged men whose body weight and mean arterial blood pressure data are collected and tabulated (Table 14.1). Biological plausibility implies that body weight is the independent variable (x) and mean arterial blood pressure is the dependent variable (y).

We want to verify if these results might be useful to predict mean arterial blood pressure based on body weight in this cohort and possibly in other similar cohorts. First, however, we must determine if there is a hint of a relationship between both variables using a graph and to quantify it (Figure 14.1).

M. Suchmacher & M. Geller: Practical Biostatistics. DOI: 10.1016/B978-0-12-415794-1.00014-8

TABLE 14.1 Data from a Cohort of 26 Overweight Middle-Aged Men[a]

Patient No.	Body Weight (kg) (x)	Mean Arterial Blood Pressure (mmHg) (y)
1	20	80
2	30	78
3	40	90
4	50	92
5	60	76
6	70	78
7	80	86
8	90	76
9	100	108
10	110	74
11	120	85
12	130	108
13	140	110
14	150	88
15	160	90
16	170	80
17	180	118
18	20	150
19	30	89
20	40	90
21	50	75
22	60	78
23	70	108
24	80	145
25	90	198
26	100	149
Mean	**142.8**	**99.9**

[a]The purpose of presented data (body weight) is merely to demonstrate the proposed concepts in a didactic manner, even though they are clinically irrealistic.

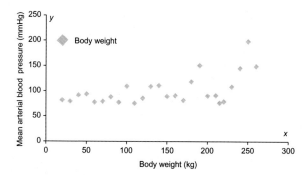

FIGURE 14.1   Scatterplot based on the data from Table 14.1.

Based on a simple visual analysis, it is possible to notice a correlation between body weight and mean arterial blood pressure variables; that is, the higher the body weight, the higher the mean arterial blood pressure. In order to better quantify this relationship, an index called correlation coefficient must be determined. One of the most commonly used is Pearson's correlation coefficient (r). This coefficient is determined by the following formula:

$$r = \frac{\sum(x - \bar{x})(y - \bar{y})}{\sqrt{\sum(x-\bar{x})^2 \sum(y-\bar{y})^2}}$$

where $\bar{x}$ is the x values mean, and $\bar{y}$ is the y values mean.

$$r = \frac{\begin{array}{l}(20 - 142.8) + (30 - 142.8) + \cdots + (100 - 142.8) \times (80 - 99.9) \\ + \cdots + (198 - 99.9) + (149 - 99.9)\end{array}}{\sqrt{\begin{array}{l}(20-142.8)^2 + (30-142.8)^2 + \cdots + (100-142.8)^2 \times (80-99.9)^2 \\ + \cdots + (198-99.9)^2 + (149-99.9)^2\end{array}}}$$

$$= +0.57$$

r ranges from -1 to $+1$ ($-$ denotes a negative direction and $+$ a positive direction). The following are possible inferences based on these data:

- The closer to 0, the weaker the correlation (dependent variable is "indifferent" to independent variable changes).
- The closer to 1 (positive or negative), the stronger the correlation (dependent variable changes as much as independent variable does).
- The closer to -1, the more the dependent variable distances from the independent variable (if the latter increases, then the former decreases, and vice-versa).
- The closer to $+1$, the more both variables change in parallel (if the independent variable increases, the dependent variable also increases).

In the previous example, $r = +0.57$. Positive direction implies two possibilities: (1) Mean arterial blood pressure is supposed to increase as body weight decreases, and (2) mean arterial blood pressure is supposed to decrease as body weight decreases.

14.2 REGRESSION

Regression (linear regression) takes correlation one step further by predicting the value of a dependent variable based on the value of an independent variable, as it quantifies the strength and direction of this prediction (the term "regression" does not imply a temporal dimension to the problem; it only represents a historical aspect of the development of this tool). Linear regression assumes that their variables present a linear relationship. This method is based on the regression line, which is determined by the linear regression formula:

$$y' = 4 + 2x$$

where y' is the value of the dependent variable to be predicted, and x is the independent variable. This means that if $x = 2$, then $y' = 8$. Graphically, this line is represented as shown in Figure 14.2.

The regression line crosses as closely as possible all the intersection points of a graph. By doing so, it is expected to represent the trend of pooled data, as well as its direction (ascending, flat, or descending line). The following are important elements of regression lines:

- Slope: Slope represents the steepness of the line. It informs on the size of the influence x has over y; that is, the steeper the line, the greater the influence.
- y-intercept: y-intercept is the point where the regression line touches the y-axis. It informs on the value of the dependent variable when the independent variable equals 0.

To predict a dependent variable, it is first necessary to build a linear regression graph by adding a regression line to the correlation scatterplot of studied population. Let us use the example from Figure 14.1 (Figure 14.3).

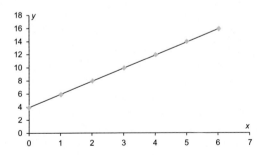

FIGURE 14.2   Regression line traced according to the intersection of independent and dependent variables.

Interpretation of a linear regression graph may depend on visual analysis (the closer to the intersection points, the greater the predictability) and biological plausibility. One can also use the linear regression formula to predict mean arterial blood pressure (y) based on any value of body weight (x) by replacing 4 for a, representing the y-intercept, and 2 by b or $-b$, representing the slope:

$$y' = a + bx$$
$$\text{or}$$
$$y' = a + (-bx)$$

where y' is the value to be predicted, a is the y-intercept, b is the ascending slope (positive direction), $-b$ is the descending slope (negative direction), and x is the independent variable.

a and b are in fact regression coefficients, which must be calculated before finding y'. Their formulas are, respectively,

$$a = \bar{y} - b\bar{x}$$
$$b = \frac{\sum(x - \bar{x})(y - \bar{y})}{\sum(x - \bar{x})^2}$$

where $\bar{x}$ is the x values mean, and $\bar{y}$ is the y values mean.

By applying the data from Table 14.1, we have the following values:

$$b = \frac{\begin{aligned}&(20 - 142.8)(80 - 99.9) + (30 - 142.8)(78 - 99.9) + \cdots \\ &+ (90 - 142.8)(198 - 99.9) + (100 - 142.8)(149 - 99.9)\end{aligned}}{(20 - 142.8)^2 + (30 - 142.8)^2 + \cdots + (90 - 142.8)^2 + (100 - 142.8)^2}$$
$$= 0.235$$

$$a = 99.9 - (0.235 \times 142.8) = 66.2$$

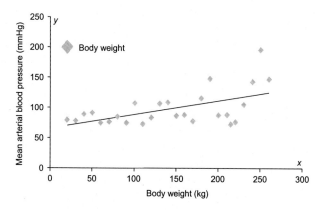

FIGURE 14.3   Regression line traced on the scatterplot from Figure 14.1.

Suppose we want to predict mean arterial blood pressure for a particular subject from our cohort. His weight is 129 kg:

$$y' = a + bx$$
$$y' = 66.2 + 0.235(129) = 96.5 \text{ mmHg}$$

Nevertheless, it is also necessary to determine how much this mean arterial blood pressure (y') is explainable by his body weight (x), according to this model. This is achievable through coefficient of determination (R^2):

$$R^2 = r^2$$

where r is the Pearson's correlation coefficient (read as "r two").

$$R^2 = +0.57^2 = 0.32 \text{ or } 32\%$$

This figure means that from all possible reasons for the patient to present a 96.5 mmHg mean arterial blood pressure (y'), 32% can be explained by his 129-kg body weight (x), according to linear regression model.

14.3 MULTIPLE LINEAR REGRESSION

Eventually, two or more independent variables are available for predicting the dependent variable. These independent variables can be considered in combination for dependent variable estimate through multivariable analysis (Chapter 3). Plenty of tools are available for performing multivariable analysis, and we focus on multiple linear regression to demonstrate this type of resource. Let us detail multiple linear regression by extending the example used previously (Table 14.2).

By scatterplotting these data together and adding a trend line for each independent variable, we can verify that x_1 and x_2 have different effects on y, as represented in Figure 14.4.

Notice how the second independent variable, diastolic blood pressure (x_2), generates by itself a steeper slope toward greater mean arterial blood pressure values. Hence, if we want to predict mean arterial blood pressure in a more "realistic" way, it would be advisable to consider both independent variables combined. If the investigator decides to do so, he or she will have two options according to the presence or the absence of interaction between (or among) independent variables:

- Independent variables do not interact.

    In this case, the multiple linear regression formula can be directly applied. With this resource, the dependent variable tends to change linearly (i.e., proportionally) with the weighted sum of independent variables. In the multiple linear regression formula, partial regression coefficients — $b_1, b_2, \ldots b_k$ — are used instead of regression coefficients:

    $$y' = a + b_1x_1 + b_2x_2 + \cdots + b_kx_k$$

TABLE 14.2 Data from a Cohort of 26 Overweight Middle-Aged Men Considering Diastolic Blood Pressure as a Second Independent Variable

Patient No.	Body Weight (kg) (x_1)	Diastolic Blood Pressure (mmHg) (x_2)	Mean Arterial Blood Pressure (mmHg) (y)
1	20	90	80
2	30	82	78
3	40	99	90
4	50	99	92
5	60	80	76
6	70	82	78
7	80	95	86
8	90	80	76
9	100	110	108
10	110	80	74
11	120	89	85
12	130	115	108
13	140	120	110
14	150	100	88
15	160	100	90
16	170	90	80
17	180	129	118
18	20	160	150
19	30	99	89
20	40	100	90
21	50	85	75
22	60	88	78
23	70	118	108
24	80	153	145
25	90	202	198
26	100	180	149
Mean	142.8	108.6	99.9

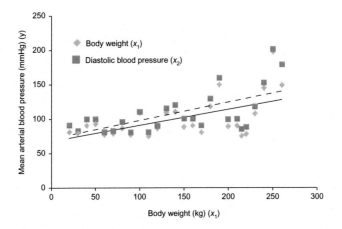

FIGURE 14.4   Regression lines for two independent variables, x_1 and x_2, traced on a scatterplot built for Table 14.2 (the continuous line represents x_1, and the dashed line represents x_2).

where y' is the value to be predicted (dependent variable), a is the y-intercept, b_1 is the partial regression coefficient to x_1, x_1 is the independent variable 1, b_2 is the partial regression coefficient to x_2, x_2 is the independent variable 2, b_k is the partial regression coefficient to x_k, and x_k is a given independent variable.

In this setting, changes in one independent variable, such as x_1, change y' on its own and not through indirect influence on other independent variables. In medical sciences, this situation represents a minority of cases, and the current example is no exception.

- Independent variables interact.

In the previous example, body weight and diastolic blood pressure — our so-called "independent" variables — are in fact mutually influenced. It is known that patients with an elevated body weight are prone to present a higher diastolic blood pressure. Therefore, body weight would be an "independent variable" to diastolic blood pressure, now the "dependent variable." In this scenario, application of the multiple linear regression formula cannot be directly performed. Partial regression coefficients must be mathematically adjusted according to the influence strength of the so-called independent variables on other independent variables that these coefficients represent (method detailed elsewhere). This strength must be statistically validated before including adjusted partial regression coefficients in the analysis. In medical sciences, this situation represents the majority of cases.

APPENDIX 14.1: HOW TO BUILD A SCATTERPLOT AND TO ADD A TREND LINE USING MICROSOFT EXCEL

Step 1

Tabulate your data, and select them disregarding subject identification and column names. Click on the **Insert** tag and then on the **Scatter** button in the **Charts** area. Select **Scatter with only Markers**.

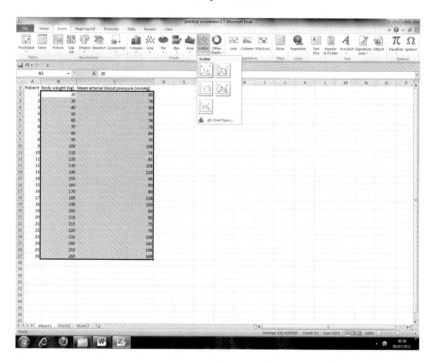

Step 2

Select **Vertical (Value) Axis Major Guidelines** and **Series 1** box (both not illustrated). Hit the delete key.

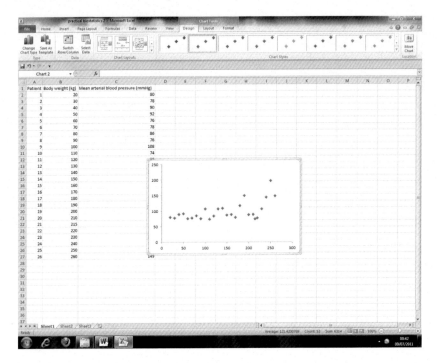

Step 3

Click on the **Layout** tag and then on the **Axis Title** button in the **Labels** area. Click on the **Primary Horizontal Axis Title** drop-down menu button and then on the **Title Below Axis** secondary drop-down menu button for the horizontal axis title box. Add desired title.

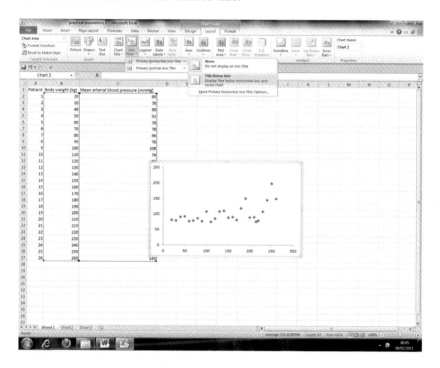

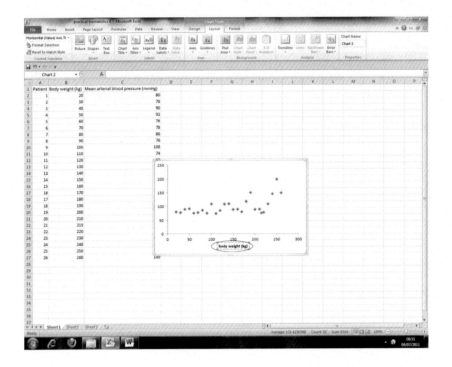

Click on the **Primary Vertical Axis** drop-down menu button and then on the **Rotated Title** secondary drop-down menu button for the vertical axis title box. Add desired title.

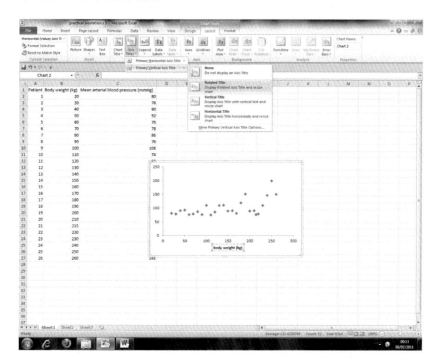

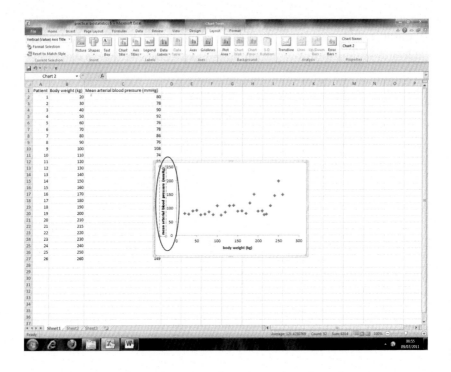

Patient	Body weight (kg)	Mean arterial blood pressure (mmHg)
1	20	80
2	30	78
3	40	90
4	50	92
5	60	76
6	70	78
7	80	86
8	90	76
9	100	108
10	110	74
11	120	
12	130	
13	140	
14	150	
15	160	
16	170	
17	180	
18	190	
19	200	
20	210	
21	215	
22	220	
23	230	
24	240	
25	250	
26	260	

Step 4

Select the chart you have created, click on the **Layout** tab, and then click on the **Trendline** button in the **Analysis** area. Click on the **Linear Trendline** button in the drop-down menu. The trend line is shown on the chart.

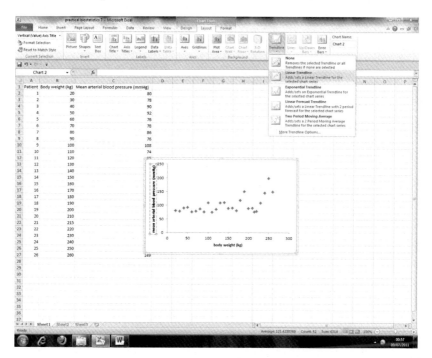

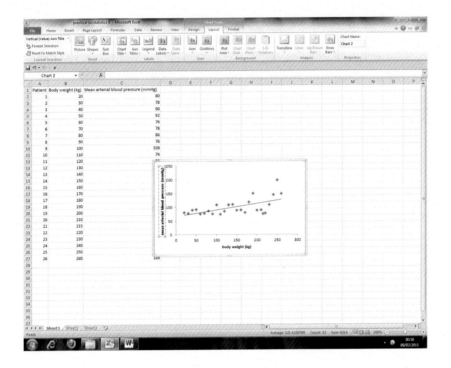

APPENDIX 14.2: HOW TO CALCULATE PEARSON'S CORRELATION COEFFICIENT USING MICROSOFT EXCEL

Step 1

Tabulate your data and select the cell immediately inferior to the columns of arguments for which you want to calculate Pearson's correlation coefficient. Click on the **Formulas** tag and then on the **More Functions** button in the **Function Library** area. Click on the **Statistical** drop-down menu button and then on the **PEARSON** secondary drop-down menu button for the **Function Arguments** dialog box.

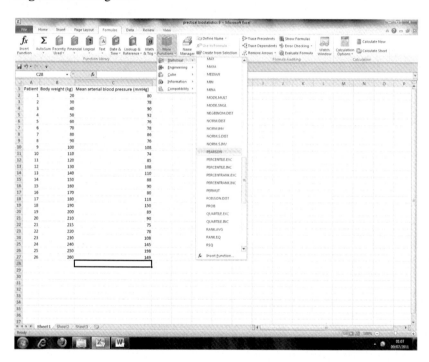

Step 2

Pearson's formula is shown in the C28 cell. Put your cursor in the **Array 1** field and then select the independent variables array (B2:B27) on the sheet itself. The array is shown in the **Array 1** field. Put your cursor in the **Array 2** field and then select the dependent variables array (C2:C27) on the sheet itself. The array is shown in the **Array 2** field. Pearson's correlation coefficient is shown in the result space.

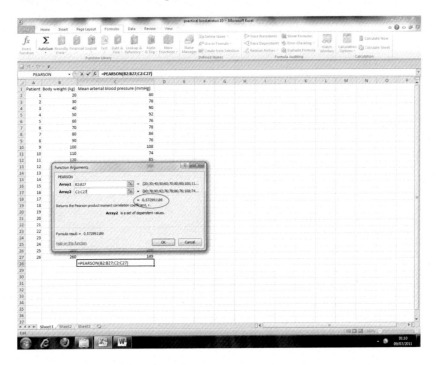

APPENDIX 14.3: HOW TO PREDICT A DEPENDENT VARIABLE USING MICROSOFT EXCEL

Step 1

Tabulate your data and select the cell immediately inferior to the dependent variable column. Click on the **Formulas** tag and then on the **More Functions** button in the **Function Library** area. Click on the **Statistical** drop-down menu button and then on the **TREND** secondary drop-down menu button for the **Function Arguments** dialog box.

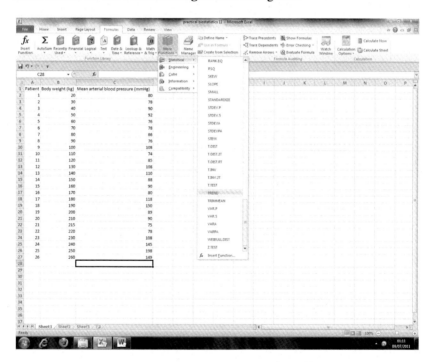

Step 2

TREND formula is shown in the C28 cell. Put your cursor in the **Known_y's** field and then select the dependent variables array (B2:B27) on the sheet itself. The array is shown in the **Known_y's** field. Put your cursor in the **Known_x's** field and then select the independent variables array (C2: C27) on the sheet itself. The array is shown in the **Known_x's** field. Leave the **Const** field blank. The dependent variable is shown in the result space.

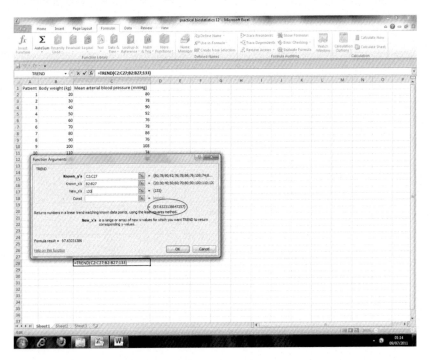

Chapter 15

Per Protocol Analysis and Intention to Treat Analysis

A research team is expected to strictly adhere to a randomized study protocol. However, although the research subject may have been fully oriented regarding his or her role, occasionally he or she can fail to comply with the instructions during the trial. In fact, investigators have poor control over this phenomenon because the research subject, after leaving medical visit and returning to daily routine, will be as subject to failures as in any average medical treatment (forgetfulness, self-neglect, and nonadherence to study visits).

This situation causes a significant dilemma for the research team, which will be forced to choose one of the following approaches for final analysis of study results, both of which have advantages and disadvantages:

- Per protocol analysis
  - In per protocol analysis, investigators are absolutely strict regarding a subject's adherence to study protocol.
    - Advantage
      Reliability of the study will be better preserved because errors generated by research subjects will be avoided. Therefore, all subjects who fail to strictly comply to study protocol are expected to be excluded from the final analysis.
    - Disadvantages
      - Total adherence to a prescribed therapy or medical orientation is not frequently seen in daily practice; rather, minor flaws occur that, in general, do not preclude completion of the treatment or its success. If the research team rejects this pattern, it would be alienating itself from so-called "real world" situations.
      - In randomized studies, if it is established that only fully adherent subjects should be considered for final analysis, a selection criterion would be generated, which could corrupt randomness. This situation would, in itself, correspond to a bias.
      - If only fully adherent subjects are considered for final analysis, the study n could be severely diminished.
- Intention to treat analysis
  - In intention to treat analysis, investigators assume a tolerant attitude regarding subject's adherence flaws to study protocol.

M. Suchmacher & M. Geller: Practical Biostatistics. DOI: 10.1016/B978-0-12-415794-1.00015-X

- Advantages

    Tolerating subjects' adherence flaws to study protocol – provided they are not severe flaws – may afford a more reliable forecast of what is expected to happen in the "real world," where the tested drug or vaccine will actually be used. Nevertheless, it is expected that randomization will itself evenly dilute these flaws, thus minimizing random error.

    During final analysis, randomization is protected through research subjects' maintenance in the study groups to which they were initially allocated.

    A partially adherent subject may have behaved so due to an adverse event, possibly associated with the tested drug or vaccine. By keeping him or her in the final analysis, this important information would be preserved, thus avoiding safety analysis error.

    Protocol nonadherent subjects may represent individuals who are also nonadherent in other aspects regarding their own health. Thus, by keeping them in the final analysis, generation of artifactual "sicker" or "healthier" samples, with accompanying bias, would be avoided.

- Disadvantage

    The inclusion of subjects not fully adhered to study protocol in the final analysis would move the conclusion of the study further away from truth.

It is important to establish the limit between a protocol flaw and nonadherence to study protocol (which should be characterized as a dropout). This parameter must be stated by the research team in the study protocol, based on the following suggested parameters:

- Tolerable frequency of posology flaws
- Tolerable frequency of nonattendance to study visits
- Research subjects should not miss visits scheduled for measurements of efficacy and safety endpoints

Intention to treat is therefore a trial results analysis type in which partial protocol adherence is tolerated in exchange for its respective advantages. In per protocol analysis, only subjects strictly adhered to study protocol are taken into account for final analysis.

Both intention to treat and per protocol analyses can be performed in the same study. For example, a new nucleoside reverse-transcriptase inhibitor efficacy in elevating CD4+ T cell blood count (expressed as cells/mm^3) in HIV+ patients (group A) is tested against a reference inhibitor belonging to the same class (group B). Results are detailed in Table 15.1.

TABLE 15.1 Results of CD4+ T Cell Counts (Cells/mm^3) for Groups A and B as Per Protocol and Intention to Treat Analyses

(n)	Per Protocol Analysis		Intention to Treat Analysis	
	30	39	44	45
Group A	503	702	439	490
Group B	550	608	490	600

One possible solution for the dilemma of which approach to adopt is to use both. If results coincide, the study conclusion will be strengthened. If not, intention to treat analysis might be preferable for two reasons: (1) It has better preserved randomization, and (2) in general, a type II error is safer for medicine than a type I error (Chapter 4).

Part IV Reader Resources

SELF-EVALUATION

1. Mark the incorrect affirmative regarding intention to treat analysis:
   A. Randomization is expected to dilute research subjects' flaws to study protocol, therefore minimizing error due to adherence failure.
   B. Lack of subjects' absolute adherence to protocol would move the conclusion of the study further away from truth.
   C. Only subjects strictly adherent to the study protocol will be taken into consideration for final analysis.
   D. Tolerating subjects' adherence flaws to study protocol may afford a more reliable forecast of what is expected to happen in "real world" practice.

2. Analyze the following study abstract and then answer the question.

   Systematic review and meta-analysis were performed, aiming to determine cognitive performance improvement in Alzheimer's disease with a cholinesterase inhibitor (test drug) against placebo, with Mini-Mental State Examination (score 0–30) as the study endpoint. Data from 11 studies were analyzed, comprising 3585 patients. Results shown in the following meta-analysis correspond to the outcome of a 12-week treatment period:

Study	Mean daily dose (mg)	n test drug/ placebo
Johnson et al.	40	302/300
Ho et al.	100	109/110
Norbert et al.	40	84/92
Mc Leary et al.	60	220/220
Gould et al.	90	150/134
Cruz et al.	90.	100/102
Amir et al.	60	101/94
Knusten et al.	40	50/94
Coopers et al.	50	12/13
Glick et al.	50	390/399
Holston et al.	50	280/281

POOLED ESTIMATE

Estimates with 95% confidence intervals (95% CI)

Points

Test drug worse ◄— —► Test drug better

A difference of 0.82 point (95% CI, 0.72−0.99) favoring test drug over placebo was found and considered statistically significant (p < 0.05).

Mark the correct affirmative:

A. Norbert et al.'s study had a larger weight than McLeary et al.'s study in this meta-analysis.
B. Amir et al.'s study did not attain significance for the pooled estimate calculation in this meta-analysis.
C. The sum of the effect size and weight of these studies influenced pooled estimate.
D. There was no correlation between n of these studies and corresponding 95% CI.

3. Find the correct correspondence:
   1. Likelihood ratio
   2. Positive predictive value
   3. Post-test odds
   4. Pretest probability
   5. Sensitivity
   a. Aggregate indexes of sensitivity and specificity
   b. Diagnostic significance index, which determines the proportion of individuals presenting a positive test result who actually have the suspected condition
   c. Index that determines the capacity of a test to detect individuals with a condition from a population in which all individuals have it
   d. Odds of an individual who presents a positive test result of actually having the suspected condition
   e. Determines the proportion of individuals with a condition in relation to a population at risk

   A. 1−a, 2−b, 3−d, 4−c, 5−e
   B. 1−a, 2−b, 3−d, 4−e, 5−c
   C. 1−b, 2−d, 3−e, 4−a, 5−c
   D. 1−d, 2−b, 3−e, 4−c, 5−a

4. Read the following study abstract and then answer the question.

   Acute bacterial osteomyelitis is a well-known complication from exposed bone fractures, and some prophylactic procedures have been practiced and tested during the past 30 years. The aim of this double-blind study was to test prophylactic antimicrobial efficacy of absorbable antibiotic-impregnated beads, associated with local surgical care. A sample of 309 patients with tibia open fracture seen in the ER was randomized: (a) 152 patients to absorbable antibiotic-impregnated beads and (b) 157 patients to absorbable non-antibiotic-impregnated beads. Clinical (local swelling and tenderness, degree of pain, and fever) and radiologic (bone erosion signs on CT) endpoints were evaluated after 21 days. Fifteen patients from the group of absorbable antibiotic impregnated *beads, and 29 patients from the group of absorbable non-antibiotic-impregnated beads, showed both clinical and radiologic evidence of marrow infection at the end of evaluation period, and the difference was considered statistically significant (p < 0.05).*

What would be the number needed to treat (NNT) for this absorbable antibiotic-impregnated beads device:

A. 10
B. 6
C. 15
D. 17

5. Refer back to the abstract in Question 4. Mark the incorrect affirmative:
   A. Changes in basal risk for acute bacterial osteomyelitis in the control group would not influence NNT.
   B. If the absorbable antibiotic-impregnated beads had been used in the control group, it would be necessary to treat *x* patients (options A, B, C, or D from question 4) so that one of them did not present acute bacterial osteomyelitis.
   C. NNT corresponds to the number of patients with recent tibia open fracture who should be treated with absorbable antibiotic-impregnated beads so that one of them benefited from the treatment.
   D. The main use of NNT is to make the probability for a successful treatment more comprehensible for physicians and patients.

6. Mark the correct affirmative regarding correlation and regression:
   A. Correlation aims to determine the degree of mathematical correlation between two variables.
   B. Correlation, as expressed by Pearson's correlation coefficient, does not influence result interpretation of regression.
   C. A dependent variable corresponds to a biological variable that has influence on another susceptible biological variable.
   D. Regression permits predicting the value of an independent variable from a known dependent variable.

7. Mark the option corresponding to a possible alternative when it is not advisable to perform a meta-analysis after a systematic review:
   A. To keep the research as systematic review only
   B. To perform subgroup meta-analysis—that is, to subdivide clinical trials pool into two homogeneous groups and then perform meta-analyses separately
   C. To perform sensitivity analysis—that is, to decrease the degree of heterogeneity among clinical trials and then try to perform meta-analysis again
   D. All of the above

8. Read the following study abstract and then answer the question.

Sensitivity and specificity of noncontrasted MRI imaging for cerebral infarct detection were studied in a sample of 82 sickle cell anemia (HbSS) pediatric patients with signs of neurocognitive impairment (measured according to Intelligence Quotient scoring) attributed to "silent" cerebral infarct. Results are displayed in the following table:

	Patients With Cerebral Infarct	Patients Without Cerebral Infarct	Total
Altered noncontrasted MRI	26	14	40
Normal noncontrasted MRI	13	29	42
Total	39	43	82

Mark the correct affirmative concerning the previous results:
A. Noncontrasted MRI has a 66% probability of not detecting cerebral infarct in a sickle cell anemia patient with neurocognitive impairment who actually does not have infarct.
B. Noncontrasted MRI has a 70% probability of not detecting cerebral infarct in a sickle cell anemia patient with neurocognitive impairment who actually does not have infarct.
C. Noncontrasted MRI has a 64% probability of detecting cerebral infarct in a sickle cell anemia patient with neurocognitive impairment who actually has it.
D. Noncontrasted MRI has a 66% probability of detecting cerebral infarct in a sickle cell anemia patient with neurocognitive impairment who actually has it.

9. Mark the incorrect affirmative:
A. Correlation aims to quantify the degree of connection of a pair of variables, and regression aims to predict the value of a dependent variable based on the value of an independent variable.
B. In multiple linear regression, independent variables are not mutually influenced.
C. The steepness of the slope in a regression line informs on the influence that the independent variable has over the dependent variable.
D. All of the above.

ANNOTATED ANSWERS

1. C. Actually, intention to treat analysis is a trial analysis type in which partial protocol adherence is tolerated in exchange for its respective advantages (resemblance to "real world" practice and avoidance of excessive *n* reduction). On the other hand, per protocol analysis rules out from final analysis any subjects who did not strictly adhere to study protocol.

2. C. In fact, McLeary et al.'s study had a larger weight than Norbert et al.'s study because the former shows a larger block and a shorter 95% CI line. Amir et al.'s study did attain significance for the pooled estimate calculation because it did not touch the "line of no effect." As a general rule, the larger the n, the narrower its corresponding 95% CI. The sum of the individual effect sizes and weights of primary studies do influence pooled estimate according to the following formula:

$$\text{Meta-analysis weighted mean} = \frac{\sum T_i W_i}{\sum W_i}$$

where i is the individual study, T_i is the effect size attributed to i primary study, and W_i is the weight attributed to i primary study.

3. B.

4. A. NNT is calculated by the following formula:

$$\frac{1}{\text{ARR}}$$

Absolute risk reduction (ARR), on the other hand, is determined by the difference between the undesired event rate in the control group and in the experimental group:

$$19\% - 9.8\% = 9.2\%$$

The inverse of 8.2 is 0.1. Therefore, NNT = 10 patients.

5. A. As a general rule, NNT changes inversely with basal risk (BR); that is, the higher the BR for acute bacterial osteomyelitis, the higher the expected ARR and thus the lower the NNT. Let us suppose that the BR for acute bacterial osteomyelitis in patients with tibia open fracture was higher so that the undesired event rate was, for example, 25%. ARR would be $25\% - 9.8\% = 15.2\%$. The inverse of 15.2 is 0.06 or 6 patients. Therefore, NNT = 6 patients.

6. A. Correlation does influence result interpretation of regression because the square of Pearson's correlation coefficient (i.e., the coefficient of determination) determines the probability of a regression result to be actually true. In fact, it is the independent variable that has influence on another susceptible biological variable. Similarly, regression enables prediction of the value of a dependent variable from a known independent variable, not the opposite.

7. D.

8. D. The probability of not detecting a condition in a patient who actually does not have it is more consistent with the detection index of specificity, which in this study can be calculated by the following formula:

	Patients With Cerebral Infarct	Patients Without Cerebral Infarct
Altered noncontrasted MRI	26 (a)	14 (b)
Normal noncontrasted MRI	13 (c)	29 (d)

$$d/(b + d)$$
$$29/(14 + 29) = 0.67 \Rightarrow 67\%$$

Therefore, specificity would be 67%, not 66 or 70% as in options A and B, respectively. The probability of detecting a condition in a patient who actually has it is more consistent with the detection index of sensitivity, which in this study can be calculated by the following formula:

$$a/(a + c)$$
$$26/(26 + 13) = 0.66 \Rightarrow 66\%$$

9. D.

SUGGESTED READING

Basic statistics for clinicians; 1995. Can Med Assoc J. <www.cmaj.ca>.

Bialostozky, D., Lopez-Meneses, M., Crespo, L., Puente-Barragan, A., Gonzalez-Pacheco, H., Lupi-Herrera, E., Victoria, D., Altamirano, J., Martinez, I., Keirns, C., 1999. Myocardial perfusion scintigraphy (SPECT) in the evaluation of patients in the emergency room with precordial pain and normal or doubtful ischemic ECG: Study 60 cases. Arch. Inst. Cardiol. Mex. 69 (6), 534–545.

Centre for Evidence Based Medicine. Department of Medicine, Toronto General Hospital, Toronto. <www.cebm.utoronto.ca>.

Centre for Health Evidence. <www.cche.net/default.asp>.

Cochrane Handbook for Systematic Reviews of Interventions (5.0.1). Updated September 2008. The Cochrane Collaboration, London, 2008.

Drummond, J.P., Silva, E., 1998. Medicina Baseada em Evidências: Novo Paradigma Assistencial e Pedagógico. Atheneu.

Estrela, C., 2001. Metodologia Científica: Ensino e Pesquisa em Odontologia. Editora Artes Médicas, Sao Paulo, Brazil.

Everitt, B., 2006. Medical Statistics from A to Z: A Guide for Clinicians and Medical Students, second ed. Cambridge University Press, Cambridge, UK.

Everitt, B.S., 1995. The Cambridge Dictionary of Statistics in the Medical Sciences. Cambridge University Press, Cambridge, UK.

Everitt, B.S., et al., 2005. Encyclopaedic Companion to Medical Statistics. Hodder Arnold, London.

Green, S., 2005. Systematic reviews and meta-analysis. Singapore Med. J. 46 (6), 270−274.

Hulley, S.B., et al., 2001. Designing Clinical Research: An Epidemiological Approach, second ed. Lippincott Williams & Wilkins, Philadelphia.

Jaeschke, R., Guyatt, G., Shannon, H., Walter, S., Cook, D., Heddle, N., 1995. Assessing the effects of treatment: measures of association. Can. Med. Assoc. J. 152, 351−357.

Katz, M.H., 1999. Multivariable Analysis: A Practical Guide for Clinicians. Cambridge University Press, Cambridge, UK.

Laupacis, A., Sackett, D.L., Roberts, R.S., 1988. An assessment of clinically useful measures of the consequences of treatment. N. Engl. J. Med. 318 (26), 1728−1733.

Merriam−Webster Online Dictionary. <www.merriam-webster.com>.

Montori, V.M., Swiontkowski, M.F., Cook, D.J., 2003. Methodologic issues in systematic reviews and meta-analysis. Clin. Orthop. Rel. Res. 413, 43−54.

Oliveira, G.G., 2006. Ensaios Clínicos: Princípios e Prática. Editora Anvisa.

Pai, M., McCulloch, M., Gorman, J.D., Pai, N., Enanoria, W., Kennedy, G., Tharyan, P., Colford Jr. J.M., 2004. Systematic reviews and meta-analysis: an illustrated? step-by-step guide. Natl. Med. J. India 17, 86−95.

Petrie, A., Bulman, J.S., Osborn, J.F., 2002. Further statistics in dentistry: Part 6. Multiple linear regression. Br. Dent. J. 193 (12), 675−682.

Sackett, D.L., et al., 2001. Evidence-Based Medicine: How to Practice and Teach EBM, second ed. Churchill Livingstone, Edinburgh, UK.

Sauerland, S., Seiler, C.M., 2005. Role of systematic reviews and meta-analysis in evidence-based medicine. World J. Surg. 29, 582−587.

Schmuller, J., 2009. Statistical Analysis with Excel for Dummies, second ed. Wiley, Hoboken, NJ.

Microsoft Excel 2010 Basics

Although plenty of biostatistics software packages are available, they generally demand knowledge at a graduation level, require extensive training, and can be costly. Despite the fact that Microsoft Excel (ME) is not specifically designed for the biostatistics field, it does have the following advantages:

- The vast majority of PC and Mac users already have it on their computers.
- ME is provided with basic statistics and mathematical resources for dealing with most biostatistical problems, from basic to moderate levels of complexity (which is the main focus of this book).
- It is a popular applicative, with widely available literature and human resources for knowledge and training.

The objective of this Appendix is to familiarize the reader with some fundamental resources of ME and statistics with ME, used throughout the book. To encompass the wholeness of ME capabilities is not part of this objective. Only the knowledge needed to support the general contents of the book is presented. The adopted ME version corresponds to the Microsoft Office Professional 2010 package running on Windows 7.

The reader is advised to complement his or her study findings reached through ME with a review by the supporting biostatistician, who is the most qualified person to draw definitive statistical conclusions from an observational study or a clinical trial.

A.1 STRUCTURE AND MAIN FEATURES OF A MICROSOFT EXCEL 2010 WORKSHEET

A basic ME worksheet presents as key buttons and fields (Figures A.1 and A.2).
The following are basic working characteristics and concepts of a typical ME worksheet:

- Whatever is typed on a selected cell is simultaneously reproduced in the formula bar and vice versa.

199

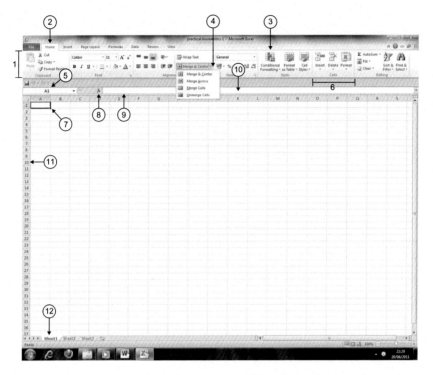

FIGURE A.1   Example of a basic ME worksheet. 1, Ribbon; 2, tag; 3, button; 4, drop-down menu button; 5, name box; 6, area; 7, cell (in this example, a selected one); 8, insert function button; 9, formula bar; 10, column; 11, row; 12, sheet tag.

- A selected cell's address is named according to a crossed alphanumeric system, with the letter representing the column and the number representing the row (in Figure A.1, the selected cell is the A1 cell).
- Any given cell's address is informed on the name box.
- The formula bar expresses the formulas applied in the **Function Arguments** dialog box and in the selected cell.

A set of symbols and terms are combined during some mathematical procedures developed on the worksheet cells, formula bars, and dialog boxes. Some of them are detailed here:

- = (equal sign)
    It points to a given correspondence or precedes a formula aiming at an objective result. For example: = 33 + 33 (Enter) → 66.
- # (number sign)
    It represents any given number.
- ! (exclamation point)
    It associates a particular sheet to a particular cell, in case you are working simultaneously in different sheets. For example: Sheet2! A2 + Sheet1!B4.

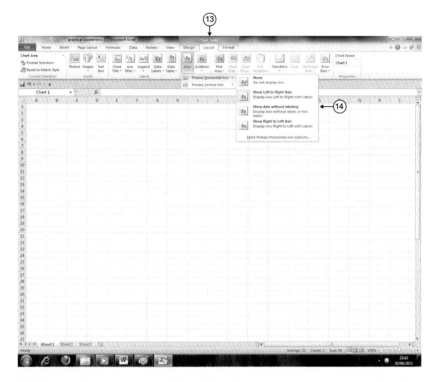

FIGURE A.2   Example of a basic ME worksheet. 13, Overtag; 14, secondary drop-down menu button.

- : (colon)

  It denotes an array of adjacent cells. For example: A1:C10 (cell A1 through cell C10).

- Negative expressions (e.g., NULL), generally followed by !

  They point out a wrong procedure—at least for that context—being performed. For example: #NULL!

- Sheet, followed by a number

  It informs you on which sheet tag you are in. For example: Sheet1.

- $ (dollar sign)

  It locks a formula or an argument to a specific cell's address or a specific array of cells. This means that whenever you refer to the former, the applicative will always direct you to the latter. For example: Sheet1!$A$1:$C$7 (the contents of A1 through C7 array of cells can only be accessed in A1 through C7 array of cells).

- ( ) (parentheses)

  A calculation from a formula inside parentheses is performed first. For example: = (B3 + B2)*3.1. (B3 + B2) will be calculated before multiplication by 3.1.

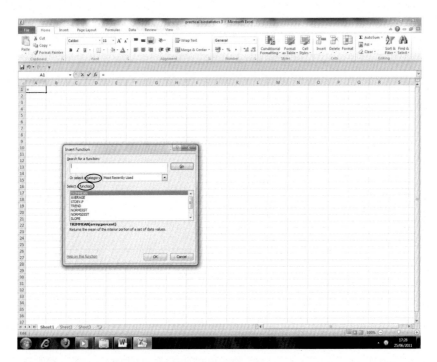

FIGURE A.3 **Insert Function** dialog box, with statistical **category** and corresponding functions shown.

category and **function** (Figure A.3) can both be accessed through the **Insert Function** dialog box (click the **Insert Function** button). A function has an implicit formula, where arguments can be inserted through the **Function Arguments** dialog box or directly in the cells. A formula has the following general components: (1) equal sign (=), (2) the chosen function in capital letters, and (3) brackets containing the cells comprehended in the calculation. For example, = SUM(C1:C8). The formula can be expressed in three different locations, most often simultaneously: (1) the selected cell, (2) the argument field in dialog boxes, and (3) the formula bar.

A.2 LOCATION OF STATISTICAL RESOURCES

Statistical functions are identified as mnemonics (e.g. standard deviation for populations = **STDEV.P**). Their working characteristics are detailed in **Function Arguments** dialog boxes (Figure A.4).

A.2.1 Basic Statistical Resources

Click on the **Formulas** tab. Click on the **More Functions** button in the **Function Library** area for a drop-down menu. Click on the **Statistics** category for a drop-down menu with basic statistical tools listed (see Figure A.5)

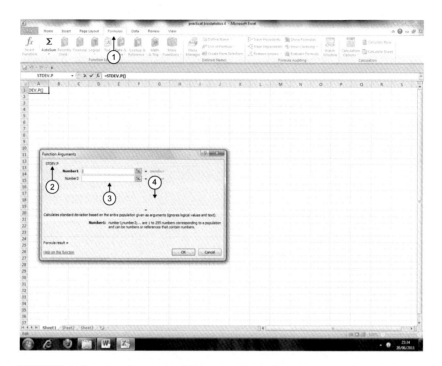

FIGURE A.4 **Function Arguments** dialog box. 1, **Formulas** tag; 2, name of the function (in this example, standard deviation for populations); 3, field for the argument or array of cells; 4, result space. Note that the formulas to be applied are expressed in the formula bar as well as in the selected cell.

A.2.2 Microsoft Excel Statistical ToolPack

To access heavier statistical analysis tools, it is first necessary to load them into Excel as follows.

Step 1

Click on the **File** tag and then on the **Options** button (see Figure A.6)

Step 2

An **Excel Options** dialog box opens. Select the **Add-Ins** option from the menu list for a drop-down menu labeled **Manage** at the bottom of the box. Select the option **Excel Add-ins**, and click the **Go…** button for an **Add-Ins** secondary dialog box. Checkmark the box **Analysis ToolPack**, and then click **OK**. Wait for loading. (See Figures A.7 and A.8).

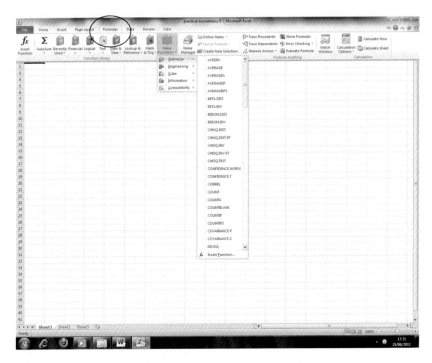

FIGURE A.5

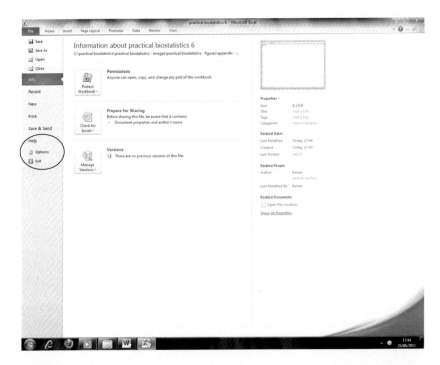

FIGURE A.6

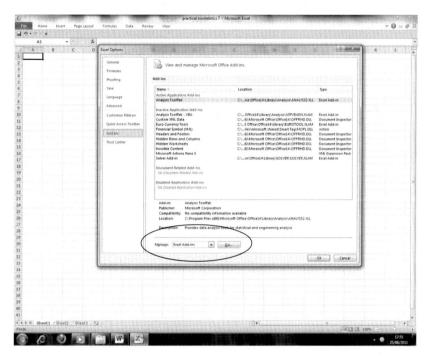

FIGURE A.7

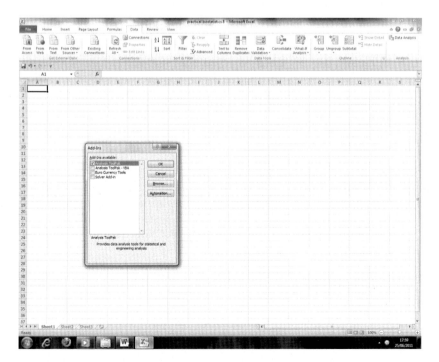

FIGURE A.8

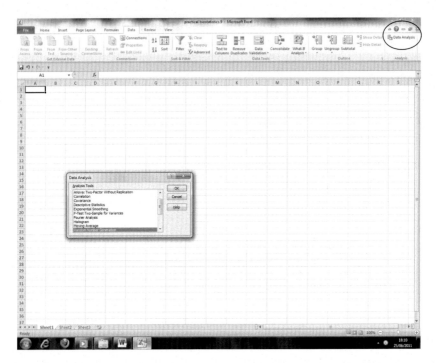

FIGURE A.9

Step 3

Check if the Analysis ToolPack was loaded by clicking the **Data Analysis** button in the **Analysis** area, located at **Data** tab. The **Data Analysis** dialog box opens (Figure A.9).

A.3 BUILDING A PLAIN TABLE

Tabulate your data with a graphic correspondence to the plain table you want to create. Select the whole array of data, click on the **Insert** tag, and then click on the **Table** button in **Tables** area for the **Create Table** dialog box. Click **OK**. An initial default table is created (see Figures A.10 and A.11).

Notice that a **Design** tab automatically opens, with five different areas underneath, as follows:

- **Properties:** allows naming the table and the insertion or exclusion of rows and columns.
- **Tools:** allows (1) expanding the table's resources with the PivotTable applicative; (2) removing duplicates from the table; and (3) removing the

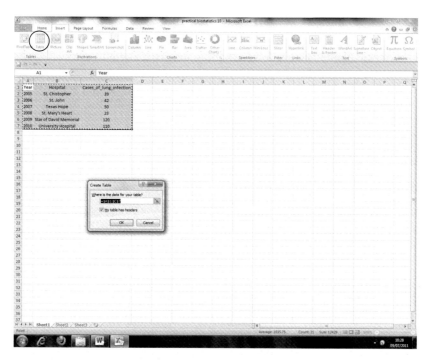

FIGURE A.10

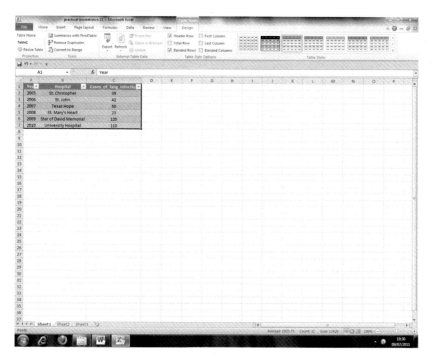

FIGURE A.11

drop-down menu from the table's header, converting it into a table with a normal array of cells.

- **External Table Data:** allows exporting the table's data to external applicatives, as well as updating them according to an external source.
- **Table Style Options:** allows visual configuration of the table.
- **Table Styles:** allows additional visual configurations for the table.

A.4 BUILDING A BASIC CHART

Click on the **Insert** tab. Then tabulate your arguments on individual cells and select the corresponding array. In the **Charts** area, there are 6 available chart types from which to choose, plus a button for 15 extra chart types. The most commonly used chart types in statistics are **Column**, **Pie**, **Bar**, and **Scatter**. We use the **Column** type (**2-D Column**) for exemplification (Figure A.12).

ME will semi-randomly assign a place for the arguments in the chart. By default, numbers are used for their identification (Figure A.13).

Notice that a **Design** tab automatically opens, with five different areas underneath, as follows:

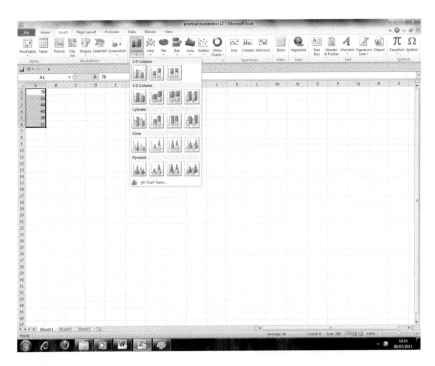

FIGURE A.12

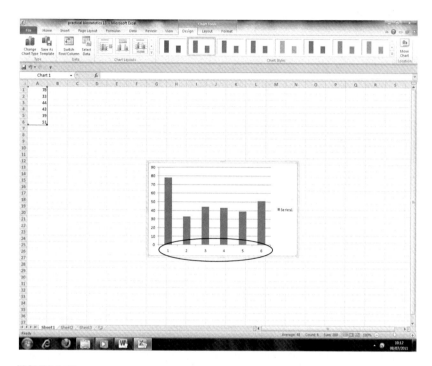

FIGURE A.13

- **Type:** Allows chart type changes and saving the chart configurations you have created
- **Data:** Allows manipulation of data between the axes of the chart
- **Chart Layout:** Allows additional graphical changes
- **Chart Styles:** Allows additional graphical changes
- **Local:** Transfers resources

An important note: Data changes on the cells are followed by automatic changes on the chart.

A.5 BUILDING A CHART OUT OF A TABLE

Let us use the table from Section A.3 and **Column** chart type (**2-D Column**) for exemplification.

Step 1

Select the array of cells corresponding to the table, click on the **Insert** tag, and then click on the **Column** button in the **Charts** area. Select **2-D Column**. A chart is shown, automatically assigned to the **Design** tab in the **Chart Tools** overtab (Figure A.14)

ME does not necessarily build a chart that precisely expresses the table's content. In most cases, adjustments performed by the user are necessary, as follows.

Step 2

There are a number of ways to adjust the graphical presentation of your chart so that it is consistent with the information expressed by the table. It is an empirical trial-and-error process in which the following tools, located at the **Design** tab, are applicable:

- **Switch Row/Column** button in the **Data** area (highlighted in Figure A.14): switches the data underneath the columns into a list disposition and vice versa. Because these data will be detached from corresponding individual columns, colors will be assigned for both for better identification (Figure A.15).
- Chart Layouts area: offers 11 different chart layouts, which might fit better to what you need your chart to express (Figure A.16).
- **Chart Styles** area: offers 48 different chart styles, which might fit better to what you need your chart to express (Figure A.17).
- Chart drop-down menus: For each aspect of the chart (the chart as a whole, horizontal axis, title, bars, etc.), there is a corresponding drop-down menu, activated by a right-click of the mouse. They offer a myriad of possibilities, according to the aspect you want to modify and to the type of chart adopted. A column drop-down menu is used for exemplification (Figure A.18).

Step 3: Naming the Chart

Click on the **Layout** tag, and then click on the **Chart Title** button in the **Labels** area for a drop-down menu. We start with the **Centered Overlay Title** button. The **Chart Title** field is inserted in the chart for you to name (or rename) it (Figures A.19 and A.20).

Step 4: Naming the Axes

Click on the **Axis Titles** button in the **Labels** area for a drop-down menu. Click on the **Primary Horizontal Axis Title** button for a secondary drop-down menu. We use the **Title Below Axis** secondary drop-down button for exemplification. The name of the primary horizontal axis is inserted in the selected **Axis Title** field in the chart. Name the axis (Figures A.21 and A.22).

Click on the **Primary Vertical Axis Title** button in the **Labels** area for a secondary drop-down menu. We use the **Rotated Title** secondary drop-down button menu for exemplification. The name of the primary vertical axis

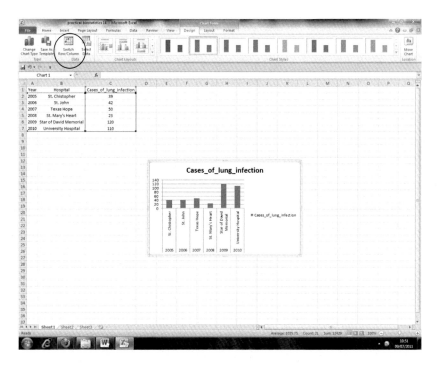

FIGURE A.14

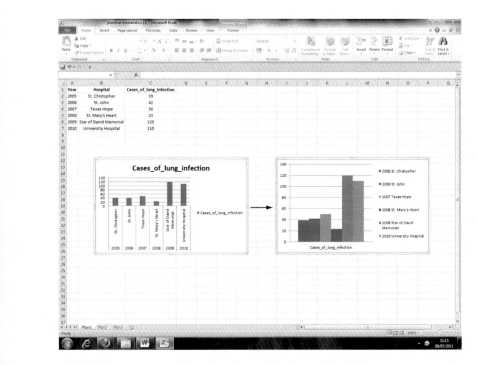

FIGURE A.15

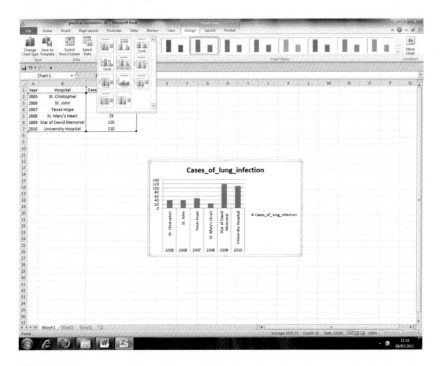

FIGURE A.16

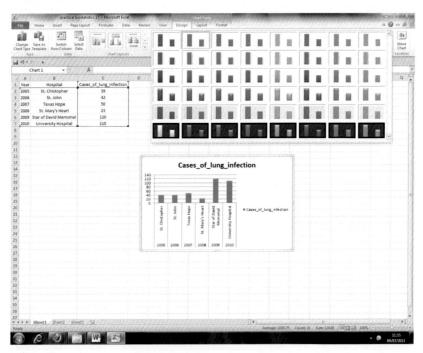

FIGURE A.17

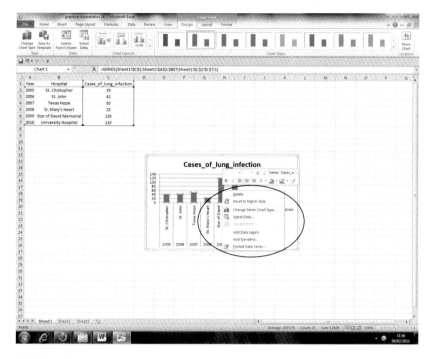

FIGURE A.18

is inserted in the selected **Axis Title** field in the chart. Name the axis (Figures A.23 and A.24).

Note that small graphical adjustments may be necessary.

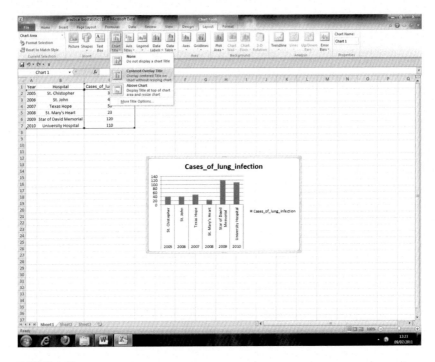

FIGURE A.19

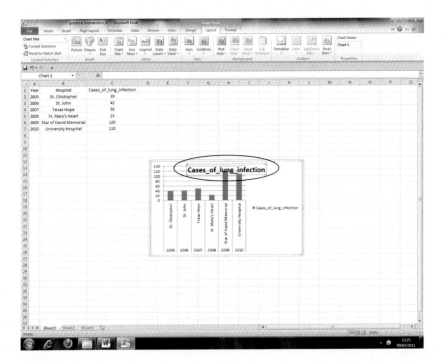

FIGURE A.20

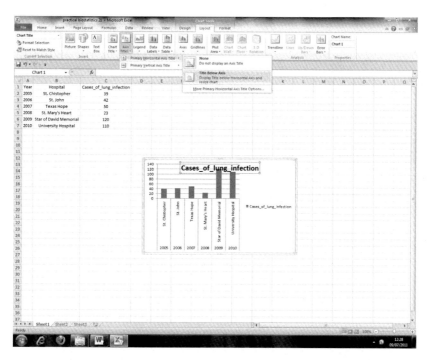

FIGURE A.21

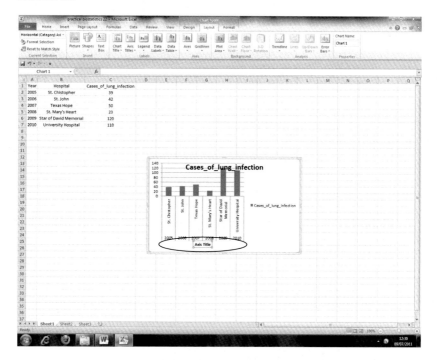

FIGURE A.22

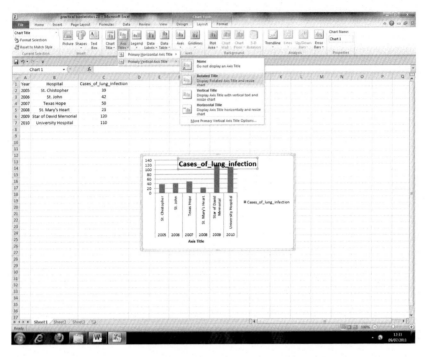

FIGURE A.23

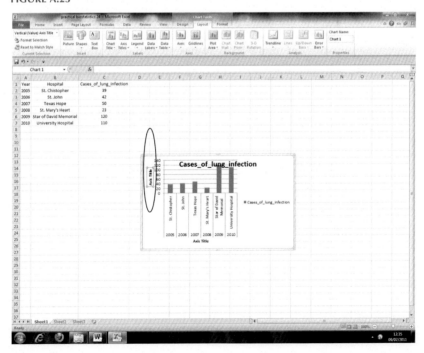

FIGURE A.24

A.6 PIVOT TABLE

A PivotTable provides tools for manipulation and cross-analysis of any amount of tabulated data. Its access path and basic structure are discussed here. (Note that PivotTable is good for a specific purpose in this book (see the appendix in Chapter 8); detailing its full resources goes beyond the scope of this book, and the reader is referred to Microsoft Excel manuals for more information.)

Step 1

Tabulate and select your data, click on the **Insert** tag, and then click on **PivotTable** in the **Tables** area for the **Create PivotTable** dialog box. Tabulated data are automatically selected, and the corresponding array is shown in the **Table/Array** field of the box. Click **OK** (by default, PivotTable is built in a new worksheet) (Figure A.25).

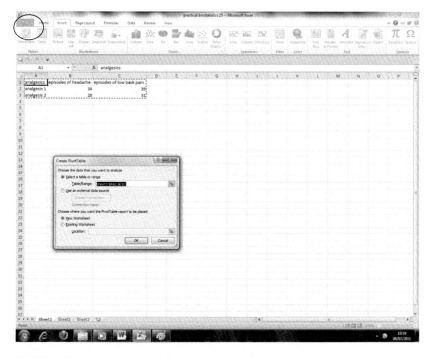

FIGURE A.25

Step 2

A PivotTable worksheet opens under the **Options** tag, and with **Field List**, +/− **Buttons**, and **Field Headers** buttons pressed. PivotTable worksheet has the following structure (Figure A.26).

- Placeholder box: instructs the user on how to create a PivotTable − here also called a "report" − by working on the PivotTable field list.
- **PivotTable Field List:** contains the tools that will allow the report buildup. It is divided into five fields:
  - Fields list: It contains the names of the columns − here also called "fields" − of the original table, with checkmark boxes.
  - **Report Filter**: It allows more refined combinations and analyses.
  - **Column Labels**: It enlists the columns belonging to the field that is dragged into it.
  - **Row Labels**: It enlists the rows belonging to the field that is dragged into it.
  - Σ **values**: It sums the values of the field that is dragged into it.

Step 3

By checkmarking fields list boxes and dragging the fields to **Column Labels, Row Labels**, and Σ **Values**, it is possible to build up a report in many different combinations for many different purposes. For example, an initial report can be built by checkmarking fields list boxes (Figure A.27).

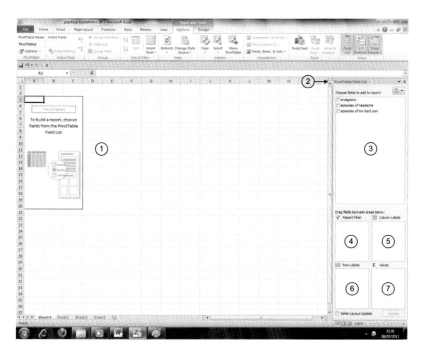

FIGURE A.26 1, Placeholder box; 2, PivotTable Field List; 3, fields list; 4, Report Filter; 5, Column Labels; 6, Row Labels; 7, Σ Values.

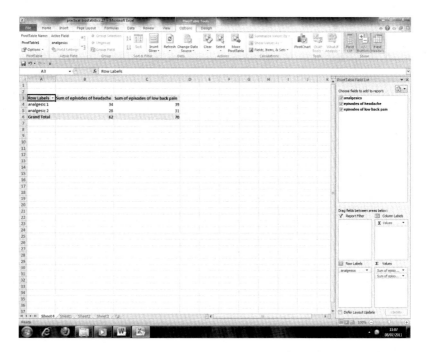

FIGURE A.27

SUGGESTED READING

Schmuller, J., 2009. Statistical Analysis with Excel for Dummies, second ed. Wiley, Hoboken, NJ. Microsoft Excel Help (Microsoft Office Professional 2010).

α   Statistical significance level that corresponds to the highest tolerable cutoff for type I error (generally 0.05).

β   Statistical significance level that corresponds to the highest tolerable cutoff for type II error (generally 0.20).

absolute risk   Probability that a disease-free subject submitted to a known exposure factor will present a given condition in a certain time span.

alternative hypothesis   Hypothesis against which antagonic null hypothesis (H_0) (see **null hypothesis**) is tested. Alternative hypothesis (H_1) normally prevails if H_0 is rejected.

argument   Denomination for a given value inserted in a cell or a formula (Microsoft Excel).

array   Two or more cells grouped together on an Excel worksheet (Microsoft Excel).

bias   Deviation of results and inferences from truth, due to systematic error (see **systematic error**).

case   A term used to refer to an individual in a population who has the condition of interest.

category   A class of Microsoft Excel formulas (e.g. statistical formulas).

chance   The possibility of a particular outcome in an uncertain situation (lexical).

cohort   Population whose individuals share common characteristics.

confidence interval   A range of values of a sample that, expectedly, contain the parameters of the general population from which it was taken, under a conventional degree of probability (confidence level).

confounder   In the context of multivariable analysis, a confounder is like a "concealed" independent variable that directly influences the dependent variable, "confounding" the investigator due to the association of the former with a more "apparent" independent variable, which in turn has no real influence on the dependent variable. For example: there is a high prevalence of high body weight (dependent variable) in a cohort of teachers of a local school. We verify that a certain brand of sweetener (apparent independent variable) is added to their coffee on a daily basis. At first, we could attribute this finding to this brand of sweetener. Nevertheless, we also verify that the coffee is inadvertently prepared with a high content of sugar (concealed independent variable, confounder) before being served to the teachers. Although this brand of sweetener is apparently accountable for the high body weight (dependent variable), it has no real influence on it but is nevertheless associated with the real influencing concealed independent variable (sugar in the coffee). This definition can be extended to contexts different from multivariable analysis.

contingency table   A table built over measured observations of a population and that cross-classifies corresponding categorical variables. A frequently used contingency table is the two-dimensional model; that is, it involves two different variables (for example, see Chapter 6).

control group   Collection of individuals used as a comparative parameter to an experimental group and tested in parallel with the latter. In observational studies, it corresponds to the collection of individuals not subjected to the risk factor.

covariate   In the context of observational studies, a covariate is a variable different from the major variables — condition or exposure — but that can also influence outcome.

critical value   Conventional cutoff value that separates statistical significance from statistical nonsignificance in a study. It corresponds to α (see α).

degree of freedom   In the context of statistics, degree of freedom (ν) is a measure of available numerical possibilities of a variable in a set of variables. For example,

$$2 + 1 + 3 = 6$$

This equation has three degrees of freedom — its first, second, and third elements — because they are "free" to vary in order to sum 6.

$$2 + 2 + z = 6$$

This equation has two degrees of freedom — its first and second elements — because they are "free" to vary. However, for this equation to sum 6, the third element, z, cannot be "free" to be any number other than 2.

dispersal   The degree to which a set of observations deviate from their mean.

drop-out   A subject who withdraws from a study for any reason.

endpoint   Efficacy variable chosen as the parameter meant to determine the outcome of a clinical trial. Endpoints can be subdivided into primary endpoint and secondary endpoint(s).

estimator   In the setting of population estimation based on sampling (see Chapter 10), an estimator corresponds to a sample statistic meant to estimate its related parameter (see **parameter**). For example, $\bar{x}$ (arithmetic mean) of a given sample — the estimator — is used to estimate μ (arithmetic mean) of the population.

evidence-based medicine   Accurate use of up-to-date and systematically harvested literary evidence; meant to support bedside decision-making processes. It is assumed that expertise on use and interpretation of biostatistical tools is fundamental for mastering this skill.

false negative   Situation in which a diagnostic test indicates that a condition is absent in a patient who actually has it.

false positive   Situation in which a diagnostic test indicates that a condition is present in a patient who actually does not have it.

f_h (fraction$_{harm}$)   See fraction$_{harm}$.

formula   Mathematical or statistical expression implicit in the function in use (Microsoft Excel).

fraction$_{harm}$ (f_h) Risk of a control patient presenting an adverse reaction relative to the risk of a treated patient.

fraction$_{treatment}$ (f_t) Risk of a control patient presenting an undesired event relative to the risk of a treated patient.

f_t (fraction$_{treatment}$) See fraction$_{treatment}$.

function A subtype of category (see **category**).

group Two or more figures forming a complete unit in a composition (lexical).

historical (literature) controls Patients treated in the past with a standard drug or vaccine who can be used as the control group (see **control group**) in a current study.

interaction In the context of multiple linear regression, an interaction occurs when an independent variable indirectly influences a dependent variable through interaction with a second independent variable. For example, suppose there is a high incidence of respiratory diseases (dependent variable) in a cohort of office employees apparently due to a low-temperature environment (independent variable) provided by air-conditioning. Nevertheless, we verify that the air-conditioning system is contaminated by a species of fungus that grows in low temperatures (second independent variable). Hence, independent variable (low-temperature environment) and second independent variable (cryophile fungus) interact. This definition can be extended to contexts different from multivariable analysis.

interval Written representation of an array − for example, A1:B10 (see **array**) (Microsoft Excel).

kurtosis The degree of sharpness or bluntness of a distribution curve in a graph.

literature controls See historical controls.

meta-analysis Statistical procedure that aims to determine efficacy or non-efficacy, generally of a medical intervention, through analysis of data across primary studies selected by a systematic review (see **systematic review**) in order to generate an average pooled estimate of their effect sizes.

n The number of individuals in a sample.

N The number of individuals in a population.

null hypothesis The no-difference pre-assumption regarding an investigator's hypothesis. Null hypothesis (H_0) is meant to be statistically tested against the alternative hypothesis (H_1), which postulates otherwise.

observation In the context of this book, it corresponds to a discrete individual or phenomenon counted in a sample or population.

odds The ratio of the probabilities of the two possible states of a binary variable − for example, the probability of symptomatic remission against the probability of symptomatic worsening.

odds ratio The ratio of the probabilities of the two possible states of a binary variable in one group relative to another − for example, probability of symptomatic remission in group A against probability of symptomatic worsening in group B.

outlier An observation that markedly deviates from the mean of a set of variables in a population or sample.

p Probability for type I error (see **type I error**).

parameter In the setting of population estimation based on sampling (see Chapter 10), it corresponds to a population variable estimated by its corresponding estimator (see **estimator**). For example, $\bar{x}$ (mean) of a given sample is used to estimate μ (mean) — the parameter — of the population.

patient expected event rate (PEER)   Expresses the proportion of patients not exposed to the putative agent and who must present the harm. It may be inferred from literary sources consistent with the potential harming agent.

PEER   See patient expected event rate.

population   In this book, this term has two meanings, depending on the context: (1) the general and broader universe of individuals from which samples (see **sample**) are taken (statistics) and (2) the total of individuals occupying an area or making up a whole (lexical).

probability   The quantitative expression of the chance that an event occurs.

random error   A study anomaly associated with a randomly erroneous parameter or process. Unlike a systematic error (see **systematic error**), the effect generated by random error can be corrected by increasing n because in the end the error will be evenly spread. For example, in a study on the efficacy of a thrombolytic drug for acute ischemic stroke, head MRIs are distributed between equally experienced radiologists A and B for diagnosis. It is expected that an eventual diagnostic error from radiologist A might be compensated by radiologist B and vice versa. It is also expected that increasing n would promote the balance between both even further.

relative risk   Measure of association between an exposure factor and the risk for a certain outcome.

risk   Possibility of incurring a loss or injury (lexical). Probability for the occurrence of an event (in biostatistics, it is often expressed as compound measures that summarize both the probability of harm and its degree of severity).

sample   In the context of statistics, a sample is a selected subset of individuals recruited from a population (see **population**).

sample size   See n.

sampling distribution   The probabilistic distribution of a statistic or a group of statistics (see **statistic**). For example, we have a population of 1000 values of a variable, from which 100 samples of 10 variables each are randomly taken, each one with its corresponding statistic. The resulting 100 statistics collection represents the sampling distribution.

sensitivity analysis   In the context of systematic review/meta-analysis, sensitivity analysis is the re-analysis of a data set oriented to determine whether changing assumptions made during a study could possibly lead to a different final interpretation or conclusion.

skewness   The degree of unilateral inclination of a distribution curve in a graph.

statistic   A variable that represents a certain statistical aspect of a sample (e.g. mean and standard deviation). Note that statistic (or its plural form) should not be confused with the term statistics (see **statistics**).

Statistics   Science concerned with the organization, description, analysis, and interpretation of experimental data.

subgroup   A fraction of a group (see **group**).

subgroup analysis   The analysis of particular subgroups in a clinical trial, often motivated by a serendipitous finding. For example, an investigator notices that a given tested analgesic unexpectedly provides better results in elderly than in younger patients and promotes a derivative analysis between both subgroups. The limitation of subgroup analysis is its propensity for generating type I errors.

surrogate endpoint An endpoint with a potential for replacing another endpoint that has a closer correlation with the study outcome but is circumstantially less convenient. For example, serum glucose levels are used rather that serum osmolarity for determining the efficacy of a new insulin formulation in the treatment of hyperosmolar diabetic coma in a facility that does not provide osmolarity test.

symmetrical distribution Frequency distribution pattern that is symmetrical around a central value.

systematic error A study anomaly associated with an intrinsically erroneous parameter or process. Differently from random error (see **random error**), bias generated by systematic error cannot be corrected by increasing n because the error will multiply itself along with n. For example, in a study on the efficacy of a thrombolytic for acute ischemic stroke, head MRIs are distributed between an experienced radiologist and an unexperienced radiologist for diagnosis. The difference between expertise levels might generate bias, and it is not expected that increasing n could correct it.

systematic review Comprehensive, protocolar, and reproducible bibliographic review of randomized clinical trials.

target population Population (see **population**) represented by a specific characteristic of interest. For example, we want to determine the efficacy of an antiviral drug for pediatric patients (population) with influenza virus infection (target population).

type I error Spurious rejection of the null hypothesis (see **null hypothesis**). For example, we state that a vasodilator is efficacious in the prevention of angina pectoris episodes when actually it is not (the null hypothesis − the vasodilator is not efficacious − was erroneously rejected).

type II error Spurious acceptance of the null hypothesis (see **null hypothesis**). For example, we state that a vasodilator is not efficacious in the prevention of angina pectoris episodes when actually it is efficacious (the null hypothesis − the vasodilator is not efficacious − was erroneously accepted).

variable A quantifiable parameter that may assume any one of a set of values − for example, body temperature, arterial blood pressure, and serum thyroxin levels.

washout A time interval introduced between two study phases in order to minimize carryover effects from the former to the next.

weighted mean An average determined through the sum of a series of different elements that takes into account their relative importance.

Index

Printed in the United States
By Bookmasters